A CHANCE FOR LIFE

The Suzanne Giroux Story

SUZANNE GIROUX
as told to Robyn Burnett

ECW PRESS

To my father, Claude Giroux, my guardian angel.
◝ Suzanne Giroux

To Jay and Amanda, for teaching me about courage.
◝ Robyn Burnett

NATIONAL LIBRARY OF CANADA CATALOGUING IN PUBLICATION DATA

Giroux, Suzanne, 1967–
A chance for life : the Suzanne Giroux story

ISBN 1-55022-449-2

1. Giroux, Suzanne, 1967– — Health. 2. Breast cancer — Treatment. 3. Trastuzumab. 4. Breast
— Cancer — Patients — Canada — Biography. I. Burnett, R.S. (Robyn S.). II. Title.

RC280.B8G57 2001   362.1'9699449'0092   C00-933260-X

Edited by Jennifer Hale
Typeset by Mary Bowness

Printed by Imprimerie Gagné / Best Book

Distributed in Canada by
General Distribution Services,
325 Humber College Blvd.,
Toronto, ON, M9W 7C3

Published by ECW PRESS
2120 Queen Street East, Suite 200
Toronto, ON M4E 1E2
ecwpress.com

This book is set in Mercurious and Minion.

PRINTED AND BOUND IN CANADA

The publication of A Chance for Life has been generously supported by the
Canada Council, the Ontario Arts Council and the Government of Canada
through the Book Publishing Industry Development Program.
Canada

Foreword

Statistics show that each year over 200,000 North American women receive the devastating news they have breast cancer. Suzanne Giroux's story is one of many.

Suzanne's story isn't just about a woman with breast cancer. It is about a woman who refused to be a statistic. She learned about her disease, pursued all available options, and, most importantly, never gave up.

While the incident rates of breast cancer continue to rise, fortunately the mortality rates have declined steadily. Every year, scientists and doctors gain a better understanding of this disease as they work to create new treatments. New drugs like Herceptin are only the beginning.

By learning more about their cancer, women can better understand what treatment options are available to them. Determining HER2 status will not only help discover Herceptin eligibility, but also can be useful in determining other possible treatments. As for prevention, early screenings, regular mammograms, self-breast examinations, and knowledge of your risk factors are avenues that could change the course of your life.

By taking control of her own health, Suzanne fulfilled new dreams that she might never have sought otherwise.

Take charge of your life; that is her message.

Suzanne's battle with breast cancer continues today.

Helen Shaver
Actor/Director/Producer

Introduction

My name is Suzanne Giroux. I was born on October 3, 1967. I was first diagnosed with breast cancer in November 1991 when I was 24 years old. I was diagnosed for a second time in September 1997 and supposed to be dead by the time I turned 31. That was three years ago.

My father, and two other guardian angels gave me a gift, a chance for life.

This is my story.

CHAPTER ONE

Father Knows Best

It all started with a 7-Up.

When he was a young man, my father, Claude Giroux, would deliver milk to the schools in Cornwall. He was a tall, broad man, with thick, dark hair and a wide smile. My mother, Huguette Bourdeau, was working as a primary school teacher on his route. A petite woman, she had curly dark hair and bright eyes. After he saw my mother for the first time, he approached her colleague, Marcel Renaud.

"God, I'd like to meet her," my father told him. Marcel revealed that my mother was a fan of 7-Up. So, the next day, instead of bringing her a glass of milk, my father brought her a 7-Up. And that was how they met.

My parents had a disciplined, religious relationship. During their courtship, they always had to ride in the car with my father's parents; my mother remembers with a laugh that they weren't even allowed to kiss. Together, they would go to the local Bingo parlour, seeing as they couldn't afford to do much else. Afterwards, they spent time together at a café sharing french fries and gravy.

My Grandfather Bourdeau only had two daughters, so he held a large wedding for my mother — over 200 guests attended! A band was hired for the event, and my mother's sister and cousin stood by her as bridesmaids.

My mother had difficulties getting pregnant. They took in two foster children before I was born: Andre and Carmen. Andre was six and Carmen was four. Their mother had left their father, and as he had no money and didn't know how to care for two children on his own, he looked for help. My parents took them in, celebrated their birthdays, and shared holidays. They became very close to Andre and Carmen, but a year later their father wanted them back. Although my parents understood the situation and believed a child should be with his/her natural parents, they were devastated. The house was suddenly very empty, and they couldn't understand why they were being denied the chance to have children. But, as God always has a plan, my mother finally got pregnant shortly afterwards.

When my mother was a young girl, her baby sister Suzanne died in her arms from a brain tumour. After such a trauma, she decided that should she be blessed with a baby girl, she would name the child after the sister she lost. So, by the time I was born, my name had been chosen: Suzanne Marie Thérèse.

It was on the evening of October 2 that my mother's water broke. Instead of going to the hospital right away, she finished watching one of her favourite television shows: *Seraphin.* Not even giving birth could keep her away from it! Finally, at nine o'clock, she checked in to the hospital. My father wasn't allowed to go in with her, so he waited through the night, pacing the hospital corridors. Suddenly, early that morning, he was paged over the hospital P.A. system. Thinking his wife had finally given birth, he rushed over . . . only to be told his car needed to be moved straight away. He ran outside to move it, and I was born at that moment — my father returned to discover he had a baby girl.

When it was time to leave the hospital, it was freezing cold outside, so they made sure I was wrapped up tight before leaving. We returned to our farm in Monkland, Ontario, to a new dilemma: the formula.

My mother wasn't breastfeeding me, so my parents debated over the specifics of my food.

"Let's give her cow's milk!" my father finally joked.

We lived on that farm in Monkland until I was four years old. It was extremely basic: no toilet, no running water. My father's sister Denise, her husband Fern, and their kids lived close by. My dad was working the night shifts at Domtar, the paper mill in Cornwall, while my mother continued on as a grade two teacher at a school in Moose Creek, where Oncle Fern was the principal. I was too young to attend school, so I kept myself entertained by spending time with my cousin Marc. His sister Sylvie was old enough to be attending school (their sister Manon would be born a few years later). Sylvie, Marc, and Manon became the siblings I would never have. My father became our designated baby-sitter, as his days were free — which for me, was perfect.

From the very beginning, I was closer to my father than my mother. He was the one who was with me all the time during the day while my mother worked. I did everything with my dad. *Everything*. Being "Daddy's Little Girl," I was always tagging along as he completed the farm chores. In the winter, when walking was difficult, Dad would keep me with him by pulling me around in a sled.

All the heavy farm labour during the day in conjunction with working the night shift at Domtar was making him exhausted. My mother was also lonely on the farm, and the lack of running water was becoming a problem. So, my parents made the decision to build a house in Cornwall, Ontario. My mother was offered a job at L'Ecole St. Lucie teaching grade two, and my father left the mill in order to work at Lalonde's, a meat market.

Cornwall is a small mill town with around 46,000 people, where nothing ever happens and everyone knows everything about everybody. A pretty area, it resides near the U.S. border, an hour from

Ottawa, and an hour from Montreal. The summers enhance the lingering sulphur smell, while the winters are harsh and unforgiving. And yet, you will always receive a warm greeting wherever you go. Tree-lined streets, with quaint cottage-like houses and friendly faces . . . it remained my home for many, many years.

We moved into my Grandmother Giroux's house on Cumberland while we waited for our house to be finished and lived there for almost a year. At the time, my Grandmother lived in a homey, two-storey house with three bedrooms, a small bathroom and living room, and a basement with a low ceiling. The house was filled with upbeat, modern furniture. My father's family had always been very open and loving, and my Grandmother Giroux was no exception.

While we were there, I had to share a bed with my grandmother. As much as I adored her, she would snore in the strangest way. I used to love to sit up in bed and stare at her lips as they wiggled. It was hard not to giggle. First, it was SNOOOORRK . . . then the slight whistle . . . WHEEEEEEE. To this day, I still ask her, "Do you still snore like that, mémère?"

The basement scared me. I hated going down into it — or any basement for that matter — because I was deathly afraid of the bogeyman. Every night, before I went to bed, I would insist that my parents check the closet *and* under the bed . . . just to make sure. And, of course, the closet door *had* to be closed tight. When I was satisfied, they would turn on a little light in the hall bathroom as reassurance. It was the only way they could get me to sleep.

Once they had left my room, I would sneak out into the hallway. On the floor, between two of the bedrooms, was a screen that looked down into the kitchen. I would curl up on the floor, peek through the little screen, and check out what the adults were up to. After a while, I would fall asleep on the floor and stay there until my dad came up to check on me. He would carefully pick me up off the floor and tuck me back into bed. Sometimes, he would snuggle up with me, singing to me in French:

"I want to live my life to the fullest. I never want to imprison it. If I feel like throwing my hands in the air, just let me, 'cause that's what I want to do . . ."

And I would fall asleep in his arms.

When I was five years old, we moved into our new home on Bruce Street. It was a typical bungalow with a huge yard for me to play in. That first day, I marched into the house with my little box and went straight into the room at the end of the hall. Back when the house was being built, I had chosen which room would be mine. It wasn't until after it had been painted and I marched in that day that we realized I'd chosen the master bedroom! But nobody argued. My mom and dad were too excited after buying a new house.

At the new house, I still spent most of my time with my father. We had a routine: I would wait after school for my father to return from work. As soon as he was approaching the house, I would quickly hide on him. He would be as tired as he could possibly be, but he'd have to find me. That was the game. I would wait impatiently, with Tiny, our chihuahua, sitting close by, wagging his tail eagerly.

"I'm right down here, Dad!" I would call quietly. And, of course, he would always find me. When he did, he'd kiss me, give me a big hug, and sit me down on his lap. Always.

The biggest punishment I ever received from my father was when I was seven. I was quite a brat at that age. My father loved gardening, and took it quite seriously. But to me, the time he spent tending his flowers was time spent away from me. So, one day, I ran around to the back yard, grabbed the hose, and sprayed him with it. He sent me to my room immediately. I'd never been sent to my room.

I waited for about ten minutes, until I heard him come around to the front of the house. As my view was right above the front garden,

I stood up on the bed and watched him through the open window.

"Daddy," I said sweetly. "You're watering the flowers, eh, 'cause they need food? 'Cause you want them to grow nice 'cause you worked really hard at it, eh?"

I went on and on. He replied with a "yup" a few times while he continued to water the garden. Finally he looked up.

"Are you hungry?"

"Yeah, I am, Daddy."

"Do you want to go to Dairy Queen and get some ice cream?"

I thought about it carefully.

"That would be hard though, 'cause I'm stuck in my room and you punished me."

"Well, come on out," he told me. And he took me to Dairy Queen. That was my big punishment.

My father moved from Lalonde's to Steinbergs, taking a job as a meat manager. The group at Steinbergs became quite close, and my parents loved spending time with them. It was a truly happy time for all of us. On occasions where my father was working, my mother and I would go on shopping excursions, and she would buy me a special lunch. Not only that, but she would pick up a little puzzle or gift for me to entertain myself with when we returned home. We began to form a bond during this time.

One weekend, Dad went on a fishing trip with the boys from Steinbergs, and a storm began brewing. My mother started getting worried, knowing my father was on the water. As the storm grew, so did our fears about his safety. She spoke to the other wives, hoping they had some news — there was nothing. We ended up waiting at one of their houses, until it was growing quite late. I was terrified at this point . . . What if he was alone in the water somewhere? *What if my father had died?*

Later that night we finally received a call from one of the men; they had made it through the fog, and found shelter on an island. It was the first time I was faced with mortality and thought I was going to lose my dad. And I realized how devastated I would be if I did.

My parents were starting to have difficulties in their marriage. My mother was still working as a teacher at this point. Her weeks went from five days, to six, and in some cases, seven. She spent so much time at the school, and hardly any at home, and my father wanted her to give it up. It wasn't just the work that was keeping her away from home, but the problems with Dad. Staying away was her method of coping with it.

Some weekends, if my father had to work, she would take me to the school with her. I tried to entertain myself in the large, empty classrooms. On occasion, I would play with the toys belonging to the different grades. Sometimes, I would draw on the dusty blackboards, making elaborate pictures. But after a while, playing by myself became lonely.

Like most young kids in that situation, I felt there was something wrong, though I couldn't really comprehend it. What I did know was that "home" wasn't a happy atmosphere. Finally, my father got fed up. He couldn't handle being alone anymore, and decided to leave.

As much as I wanted to go with my father, I didn't want to leave my house, my room, my friends, or change schools. Dad was planning on moving to a different part of the city. While I would have been able to go to school with my cousins, I had my own friends where I was. And I was afraid of the unknown. I couldn't go with him.

Dad left on August 22, 1976. He kept trying to put his suitcase in the trunk of his large, brown car and I kept trying to pull it out. I kept crying and crying, pulling at the suitcase. "Sue, please, stop it," he would say through tears, "It's hard enough as it is." I could tell my father's heart was aching.

Finally, I ran past my mother into the house and crawled under my bed. Squeezing my eyes shut, I clutched onto the big blue teddy bear that my parents had bought me for my birthday. I stayed there, crying, until my mom came to get me a few minutes later. She too, was having one of the most difficult days of her life. My father drove to his sister's house — my aunt Denise's, hoping to stay there for awhile. He had to make a few decisions. Either he was going to start a life of his own, or move back home and try to work things out.

He got an apartment.

It was a bachelor's apartment with a little closet for storage, a small bathroom, and a cramped open-concept kitchen. He bought a new wood table, a moon-shaped Venus TV and a red and black checkered hide-a-bed to sleep on. He would try to make everything as natural as possible when I would visit him on the weekends. We would spend a lot of time at Tante Denise's: it felt more normal than the apartment, and I could play with my cousins. When we did stay in, he would cook all sorts of comfort food. In the mornings, we had pancakes drenched with maple syrup. Tante Denise would give us homemade raisin bread that we smothered in peanut butter. Then, we would sit down with our chocolate milk, and watch Bugs Bunny. Dad didn't have any time for Coyote or Road Runner — it was Bugs Bunny he liked. Then, at night, I would snuggle beside him on the pull-out couch, wishing I didn't have to leave him.

My mother fell apart after my father left. She started seeing a counsellor, Pierre. Eventually, my father agreed to join her at a session, and Pierre suggested to them that divorce seemed to be the best solution. After that comment, my father stopped going. Neither one wanted a divorce, but overcoming their problems seemed too difficult at that time.

My mother stopped eating, dropping from 150 to 115 pounds. She would buy me whatever TV dinners I wanted, just so she wouldn't have to cook. Even simple things like putting on nail polish became an effort because her hands wouldn't stop shaking. She didn't show this to my father, though. She pretended everything was fine whenever he came to pick me up for the weekend. Once, after we had washed the carpets in the house, she wanted my father to believe that she had hired someone to do it. I couldn't figure out what was going on.

But it was simple. My mother was having a nervous breakdown.

It was the worst part of my childhood. Not only was I alone with my mother at home, but she was also my teacher at school. I was eight years old, and in grade two at the time, and all of a sudden, I became defiant.

"I don't write with the right hand anymore," I declared indignantly one day. "I write with the left hand."

I started refusing to listen in class. My notes were terrible. I didn't know how to read, and I spent all my time rebelling. At first, she tried putting me in the corner, but even that didn't stop me from causing problems. Finally, they had to put my desk in the hallway, because I was continually disrupting the class! Looking back, my behaviour was pretty typical of a child whose parents were getting divorced. There was no counselling for kids back then, so I didn't talk about it with anyone. While the separation was difficult for me, my poor mother had it worse. She had to deal with my antics day *and* night!

As a consequence, my mother tried to get me involved in things. Her sister's daughter, a year or two older than me, was involved with the Majorettes. So, I started to go to Majorettes every Thursday night. We wore little white skirts, little T-shirts, cowboy boots, and tights or nylons. Practices were inside and outside, preparing for the upcoming Santa Claus parade. When it was outside, I remember freezing my butt off, it was so cold! But I really enjoyed it, and it made that period of my life easier.

Dad would call up once in a while to talk to my mother. On her birthday, he called her up and asked her out for dinner Saturday night. After dinner, he slept over at the house. As the weeks passed, he would sleep over more frequently until, more often than not, he was at home with us. Finally he and my mother had a serious discussion about the situation. In order for him to return, my mother would need to spend more time with the family. She agreed.

They took me out for supper at Anchors, a romantic restaurant with candles everywhere, and informed me they were getting back together. Even though Dad had been practically living at the house, I was thrilled to know he was returning for good. Mom quit school after twenty-three years of teaching and Dad moved home just in time for Christmas. As soon as my Dad moved back home, I started using my right hand again and could read once more. My Christmas present that year was an organ, and I began learning how to play the piano.

The rebelliousness was gone.

We spent Christmas day at my Grandmother Bourdeau's. Going to Grandma's was like walking into a different world. She cooked the entire meal over an old wood stove. We would all start with glasses of homemade tomato juice and salads, then move on to the main course. And the pies! She would bake meat pies, sugar pies, apple pies. Every time I left my Grandmother's, I swore I wasn't going to eat for a week. Everything was so good and so filling.

While my parents had been separated, Dad had opened up his own butcher shop with his younger brother, Oncle Robert. Named "B & M Meat Market," it sat on the corner of Cumberland and Ninth Streets. He started selling bulk food before it became popular. Every time I would visit, I sampled a few of my favourite cookies — chocolate-covered fingers and double chocolate fudge with icing in the middle. Meanwhile, my mother started doing a lot of volunteer work at the hospital. She took care of people, cooking and cleaning for them. She also started cooking for a priest, Père Denis Vaillancourt, with whom she worked for many years.

At this point, I had gotten involved in school. I loved going because I had a lot of friends. I was always the president or the vice-president of the class, and while I never got to be the school queen, I always entered the pageant. They would begin the school Winter Carnival pageant by picking a king and queen of the classroom, who were chosen based on talent. After that, you had to compete against the whole school. I would always do my baton routine, and I'd win the classroom competition, but not the school one.

I was in grade four when I broke my foot. I had been at school playing elastics with some friends, and I twisted my ankle. The pain was terrible. The principal tried to locate one of my parents, but had no luck. Then they called Oncle Robert, hoping he could take me to the hospital, but they couldn't track him down, either. No one showed up for me until after school. I spent the day with this intense pain, just praying for someone to take me to the hospital. No one came. I sat out in the hallway with my foot swelling up, while my friends all came out to see how I was doing. I remember feeling so terribly alone. It wouldn't be the only time in my life I felt like that among friends.

That whole summer, I was in a cast. I couldn't go swimming, which was torture. And when I went to the doctor to have the cast removed, he told us it hadn't healed properly because I was using my foot too much! As a consequence of my stubbornness, I had that cast on for another two weeks. All I had wanted to do was go swimming, and by the time the cast was off, summer was almost over.

I used to love the summers because that was when we would go camping with my dad's family. In the beginning, we would travel to different camp sites. We'd gather up the whole family, and make huge barbecued suppers each night. No one could ever eat alone. All the tables would be lined up, with lots of beer passed around. Dad would hide the cooler afterwards, being cautious of the bears, while the kids would go fishing with bread, using nets to catch the minnows.

That part of my life was fantastic. Being an only child, I loved the time I spent with my cousins. While Marc and I were the same age, Sylvie was only a year older, and Manon a couple of years younger. We'd camp in the summertime and every winter we'd drive down to Florida. And whenever we could, we'd swim for hours.

I spent half my time with Sylvie and Marc in one camper, and then I'd switch over to the other camper with my parents. As we drove down south, we would stop at places on the way. I remember Nashville, because it was there I had my first taste of the gory events that could occur in hospitals. Marc and I had been in the pool all day, and he was trying to gross me out. He started recounting all the nasty details of the time he got stitches — and was especially specific when he mentioned the needle going into the wound.

"It *hurt so much*," he said, dramatically.

"Oh, my God!" I would squeal in response. He had achieved his goal.

We got called in to go and eat, so we headed back to the trailer. And, as it would happen, I was heading inside the trailer to get a chocolate pudding when . . . *SLASH*. I cut my leg on the bottom of the trailer door. Once I realized what had happened, I started screaming hysterically.

"MARC TOLD ME I'M GOING TO HAVE A NEEDLE AND THEY'RE GOING TO STICK IT IN!" Over and over again, I wailed. My father and uncle didn't know what to do. I was terrified, shaking and bleeding — and inconsolable. Marc definitely treated me like a sister, no question about that!

We had the "heavy duty" camper with the bath and shower. We also had CB radios, which we used to talk to each other as we drove. Dad was "Big Butch" while mom was "Shopping Lady." As Marc was a good student, and I wasn't particularly strong at reading, I would get him to read *all* the signs to me — all the way to Florida. Every sign was exciting when someone else was reading it.

Our family camped together up to our teenage years. Once we got older, we didn't want to hang out at the campsites anymore. We wanted to stay in town with our friends.

One of the last times we went camping, my father arranged to spend some time with me alone. He liked to know what was going on in my life, *especially* now that I was growing older and boys were becoming a factor. I was 15, and I had a thing for a guy called Tom who was three years older than me. My father knew it. So he came up with a plan. Every day, my father would take all the kids water-skiing after supper. One night, however, suddenly no one was going water-skiing. I was alone with my dad and got no explanation.

"What's going on?" I asked him.

"C'mon, we'll go fishing instead," my father answered.

"Awwwww, but I want to go water-skiing!" I complained.

He had his agenda, and I finally went along with it. Out on the boat, he danced around the topic, wanting to know certain things but never saying anything directly. The simple fact was, he wanted to know if I had kissed Tom yet.

"Okay, let's take the anchor out. Let's GO!" I said impatiently.

I pulled at the anchor, wanting to start the boat up.

"Woah, woah, woah!" he said, grabbing the keys from me. "We're going to have a father to daughter talk."

His saying was, "Father Knows Best," and he would always begin every serious discussion with that phrase. "He's too old, you're too young" or whatever appropriate response came with the point, it was always after Dad declared he knew "best." Every time. And when it came to holding on, or letting go, my father truly believed he knew best. A lot of the times, I would have to agree.

We would always take our dog Tiny with us wherever we went. He was with me throughout my childhood. He had a little routine every day when I came home from school, where he would run around the house in circles. Up and down the couch, through the kitchen, around the table, and back to the couch. Talk about a welcome home.

As he grew older, Tiny started getting sick and coughing up blood. The vet informed us he had cancer, and it was only getting worse. I knew eventually my parents were going to have to put him to sleep. I came home one day near the end, and called to him, but he didn't run to me. He was too weak. I started to cry because I knew it was time to let him go, and I didn't want to.

I hated the fact that Tiny had been put down. It took me a while to adjust to it. I would come home and get upset simply because I had been so used to his greeting. My parents could see the effect it was having on me. One day, as I walked by the closet, I heard a whimper from inside. I asked my mom what it was, and she told me to look. When I opened the closet door, I was surprised by the cutest little puppy — half German shepherd, and half Saint Bernard. We called him King, because he was perfect.

My father knew that life brought sorrow, but also joy — death does not stop life. Life goes on. Life means trying new things, taking risks, accepting the truth no matter how painful, and moving forward. It's the only way to go.

The night before the first day of high school, I spent the whole night combing my hair, testing different styles, just to make sure it would be nice for the next day. For two hours, I was on the phone with friends, trying to decide what I should wear. I didn't have a lot of clothes to choose from, which made me feel a little insecure, so a lot of the time, I would borrow clothing from different friends. I wanted to look *good*.

For me, high school was a social event. All my report cards noted that I talked too much. While I did well in gym and social studies, I had difficulties with subjects like biology and chemistry. I didn't study, which was my biggest problem. I was always on the phone, making sure I knew where the next party was. Being a social butterfly meant planning the whole weekend for me and my friends, and making sure we'd have a good time.

I was still spending time with my cousins, but in high school, it was Sylvie who I hung out with the most. We would head out to the movies or go shopping — always on the lookout for eligible young men, of course. On Saturday afternoons we would head over to Disco Wheels, hoping that we'd get asked to roller-skate to the slow songs. We had a blast. Sylvie was older than me, but it didn't make one bit of difference.

It was Sylvie's fault that I got caught smoking. I only tried it once, just a puff of her cigarette. I didn't like it. But when Tante Denise caught her, she told my father. I was so paranoid, imagining how he would react. My father was a smoker at the time, however. When he found out, he sat me down and handed me a cigarette.

"You wanna smoke?" he asked me. "Have one with me."

I coughed my brains out. He yelled at me a bit, raising his voice for only a moment, then it was done. One puff of a cigarette got me a quick talking to, and fortunately for me, that was it.

I didn't get into too much trouble in high school. I did what average teenagers did. On occasion, I would have parties at my place when my parents went away for the weekend. They would return, and the house would be cleaner than when they left. That's how it went: somebody would have a party and all four high schools in Cornwall would show up! "Lucy Smith is having a party!" "Sue Giroux is having a party!" My parents never did find out.

Chantal and Lynn were my two closest friends in school. Giggling over boys was one of our favourite pastimes. When I was in grade 10,

I had a huge crush on the boy who sat in front of me in math class: Stephane. Steph was a year older than me. The biggest clown in class, he had blond curly hair and wore bright pinks, oranges, and purples. He was a charmer, a flirt, but it was harmless. Chantal and I would pass notes back and forth all period about how crazy I was for Steph.

"Oh, my GOD, he said HI to me!" When he signed my yearbook at the end of the year, I was thrilled! But like all crushes, they eventually pass and someone new comes along.

I baby-sat the neighbourhood kids quite frequently. The whole baby-sitting thing worked well for me. I dated a guy named Tyler for a short period of time. One night, I arranged for him to pick me up when I was finished with the kids. My father thought I was still baby-sitting, as I told Dad this was a night that the kids' parents were coming home *really* late. I thought, "Hey! I'm going to get away with this one!"

Well, later my father called the house where I baby-sat only to discover I wasn't there. So, he waited quietly in the dark for me to return. Tyler took me home, and I felt reassured — the house was still dark. We started necking at the side of the house when, all of a sudden, my father came out, turned on the porch lights, and confronted us.

"What do you think you're doing, young lady?"

I choked. Tyler looked terrified.

"Um, Dad . . . this is Tyler," I squeaked.

Tyler quickly hopped into his car and took off. I waited for Dad to speak.

"Get in the house," he ordered.

As usual, my father never stayed angry with me for long. Things would go back to normal pretty quickly. In the mornings, I would play the album *Syncronicity* by the Police as I got ready. My father loved it. He would always shout from the bathroom, asking me to replay the album, singing along as he shaved. On Sundays, my father would convince me to go to church by bribing me with a beautiful breakfast afterwards — but only if I went. As we got prepared to leave for mass, my mother would find an evangelical station to watch on television. Not only did we have to go to church, but we also had to watch it for the rest of the day!

The one time I thought my father would never forgive me was after I rolled his van. I was 16 years old, and it was the first week after I got my license. I wasn't drinking, it was just a stupid, stupid thing. That night, I was baby-sitting with my friend Danielle, and we called our boyfriends up. My boyfriend, Barry, was at a party down the road, so I asked my Dad if I could borrow his van and head over to the party when I was done working.

"What time does everyone else have to be home at?" he asked.

"One," I said.

"For you, 12:00," he said.

That was fine by me because we both knew I'd come back at one anyway. I would fix my watch by setting it an hour back. I'd done that a few times. It worked for a while, until my father declared that it wasn't going to work anymore.

As we were driving towards the party, we reached a corner. As I turned, I must have turned too sharply, because suddenly, the van was rolling. While I never got charged for it, I was terrified of my father's reaction. We were right next to a field, and all I wanted to do was run — run through the field as far as I could, just to make it go away. But I stood there, awaiting the inevitable. When my father got there, he didn't get angry with me. His only concern was that I was okay. I was so embarrassed and hurt for what I had done to him. People around school would talk, as they do, and I remember feeling stupid and insecure. I couldn't hold my head up for a long time. My friends were worried, wondering if I was okay. The fact was, I was afraid of what other people thought. And I was mostly concerned with what my father thought of me.

I met my first real love, Ron Maynard, soon afterwards. He was a college boy — tall, dark, handsome, and most importantly, older! We met through my best friend, Lynn. Lynn and I had a habit of dating best friends. When she started dating a college boy, Mike, she suggested a blind date for his friend Ron and I. So, Lynn and I went off to watch Mike and Ron play in a hockey game. Afterwards, a group of us headed over to Bojangles, a local pub. We were too young to get in, but Ron knew the bouncer at the door, and he let us in. Nowadays, it's not quite that simple.

Upon first sight, I had decided that Ron was indeed cute. We hung out there for a while, then headed back to Mike's place for some of his mother's famous spicy hot spaghetti. There was another guy with us, Larry, who was also showing some interest in me. Finally, Ron pulled me to the stairwell and laid it on the line.

"Okay, I've had enough. Pick which one you like best."

So I chose him.

Ron fit well into my life. He became my "Pookie Bear." He had a large family that welcomed me with open arms. I spent a lot of time at his house rather than at mine, which saddened my father. In the mornings, Dad would drop me off at Ron's so that Ron could drive me to school. What he didn't know was that Ron's mother had already left for work. I missed a few classes on occasion seeing as *"Monsieur"* was a *college* boy, and his classes started later! He would drive me to school in his brother's orange and white Camero convertible.

I had started working in the cosmetic department at Jean Coutu Pharmacy by this time. I became close with the girls there, chatting away with the different departments over the phone system. After work, we would spend lots of time at our regular pub, Movieola's. One of the girls was a few years older, so she would sneak us all in while Ron would act as the designated driver for the night. We would dance the nights away! The waitress knew us so well, she would come out on the dance floor to get our drink orders. As the night went on, we would even get up on the speakers to dance!

Ron got along just fine with my other friends as well. One weekend, we all went up to Chantal's grandmother's cottage to spend the day there. We went canoeing, paddleboating, fishing — you name it. Then we started preparing for the barbecue dinner. As Ron was cutting up the ribs, I started getting a little flirtatious with him. I grabbed his side, and the knife accidentally hit my arm. It only touched the skin, but as the knife was so sharp, it cut through. There was a big panic, and a big rush to the hospital . . . as well as blood all over the place. Ron kept saying, "You don't need stitches" over and over. But I did need stitches. *Stitches!*

Boy, was I screaming his name across the hospital. He was no Pookie Bear there. The majority of our relationship was accident free, however.

I spent my time enjoying my last years of high school. My babysitting years had ended, as I was more interested in going out on Friday nights than staying in and watching *Dallas* or the *Dukes of Hazzard*. We'd go to a lot of school dances, and we'd also have large bonfires in my backyard. We had an in-ground swimming pool built, and I would have all my friends over for pool parties. My mother would cook up large spaghetti meals, while my Dad would always join us for a couple of beers. (Truth was, I think he loved it when all the girls hung out in their bikinis!) After the bonfire was over, we'd head to the pool. Dad would be inside, watching through the window to make sure nothing funny was going on. Skinny dipping in "Sue's pool" became a common pastime.

I had stopped keeping a diary, because I was worried my mother would start looking through it. She did find my birth control pills, however. I was 18 years old, and I thought being on the pill was much better than having a child. I tried to explain that to her, but she wouldn't hear it.

"It's not *Catholic!*" she cried. "You aren't supposed to be *doing that!*"

There was no resolution in sight. I was sure my Dad knew, and I knew he could understand — as much as he couldn't. One time, he actually caught us. He didn't say anything to me until after Ron left that night. Then he made an offhanded comment about it.

"What?!" I said, mortified, "WHAT?! OH MY GOD, WHAT WERE YOU DOING? SPYING ON ME?! CHECKING ME OUT?!"

"No," he replied, calmly. "I just wanted to go down to the basement and get some wood, and . . . well, then I thought I should just come back upstairs."

That was the most we ever said about my sex life.

I hung out with Lynn and Chantal until the end of high school. As the summer would approach, we would occasionally skip classes. One beautiful summer's day, Chantal and I skipped French. We were sitting outside by the side of the school, and our local newspaper, the *Standard Freeholder* came by. They asked to take a picture of us, and we agreed, thinking it would be cool to be in the paper . . . until we realized we'd have an interesting time explaining why we were outside rather than in class! Chantal's uncle was the vice-principal of our high school, and the next day we got called down to the office.

"And exactly what time of day was this picture taken?"

"It was our spare! It was our spare!" we pleaded.

But they caught on. We sat, squirming in the principal's office, but giggling and laughing at the same time about how stupid we had been. We couldn't just *sit* outside, we had to get the *Standard Freeholder* to take a picture of us! Skipping school and photographed. Not good.

I was at a point where I had to decide what I wanted to do when I graduated. But I had no idea. I went to see the school counsellor and wrote a test, hoping to find out what it was that I would be good at. My personality fit things like nursing, dental assistant, and so forth.

So, as the students had to pick three places to apply to, I chose nursing college, dental hygiene college, and the police academy. The third was the funniest. Nursing came in first. The college was located in Cornwall, which my parents loved but I didn't. Ron had started working in Ottawa by this time, so of course, that played a role in my decision. Dental hygiene was in Ottawa, so the decision was made.

I loved Ottawa, but we came home almost every weekend. I didn't like where I had ended up living. I had agreed to share an apartment with Chantal, but within a week, she had moved back home. She hadn't even finished high school yet, and her boyfriend was in Cornwall. After she left, I called up Ron at work, crying on the phone.

"I'm all alone! I'm lost!" I cried.

"What's wrong? What do you mean?"

"Chantal's left! Chantal left and took all her furniture!"

Everything was cleared out. Ron came over, and we had a couple of drinks. Then, he took me to a Huey Lewis concert. I had a great time — it was a fantastic concert just outside the city centre. Afterwards, we ended up partying with some friends of his in Hull, Quebec. After a short ride in a pick-up truck, we walked home in the rain. We ended up kissing on the sidewalk under a tree because the rain started falling too hard. Ron and I had our share of romantic moments.

I ended up renting another room from a woman, which I hated because I felt so alone. Fortunately, I spent most of my time with Ron, which meant I wasn't there that often. It was hardest at night. I wasn't comfortable in the house, and because of that, I made Ron stay on the phone with me on occasion until I fell asleep.

"Still there?" I'd ask, sleepily. "Still there?"

"Hang up the phone, Sue. Go to bed now," he'd say.

"No! NO!"

I didn't really hang out with too many people at college, except for a couple of girls. It was my own fault. I missed out on the social aspect of college because I was going out with Ron, but by no means do I regret it. It was after I was done with school and had moved back to Cornwall that I started hanging out with the friends I made at college. College lasted for one year, and I returned home.

Back then, I couldn't afford to keep my apartment in Ottawa and I didn't even think of moving in with my boyfriend. I was 19. If I had moved in with Ron, my father would have shot me. Not only that, but Ron and I were on the rocks. Just before I returned home, Ron finally broke it off. The long distance was too much. And because I was coming back to Cornwall and he was staying in Ottawa, I felt insecure. So, we reached the end.

Telling my parents about my break-up with Ron was one of the hardest moments in my youth. I thought I'd never survive it; he was the love of my life. I stayed up so many nights just crying inconsolably. In the middle of the night, my mother would get up and join me, making me Habitant pea soup because I hadn't eaten all day.

I started working right away when I came back here. My first step was to send résumés to all the dentists in town. Once I had stuffed all the envelopes, I realized there was one envelope that didn't have a stamp. It was for Dr. Jean and Luc Leboeuf's office.

"Well," my mother said, "I'd better go get you a stamp for that one because . . . you never know."

She was right.

I went in for my interview with Dr. Leboeuf. I hadn't completely moved back into town yet, or had my graduation party. And Jean said: "Well, you want the weekend?" "Okay," I squeaked. I was hoping to have a couple of weeks after college, but I would be starting work that Monday.

At work I made sure I had fun. I had become friends with Rita, another dentist at the office. I was also working closely with Joanne Pilon, a girl I had been friends with in high school who had become a dental hygienist. Rita was living alone, and had nothing to do at night, and Joanne had grown up close to me, so we started hanging out. When we would pull wisdom teeth out together, we made a game of it. If it had two roots, I would whisper: "Oooooh! It's a baby girl!" Three roots, and it was a baby boy. I would declare it quietly so only she could hear, and we would break into giggles.

Now that I was single, I was having a lot more fun with my girl-friends. It got a little hectic living at home, though. It wasn't too long afterwards that I met Steve. He was on a blind date with a girlfriend of mine, and she didn't like him! I thought she was nuts.

"You don't want him? I'd like to meet him!" I told her.

So the next time we got together she introduced him to me, "Here! Meet Sue!" We hit it off immediately.

Steve and I were engaged for a short time, but it didn't last. The problem was, he played baseball all the time, and his friends were his life. When we were still together, however, his father passed away. It was winter, and his father was dying in a hospital in Kingston. We got in the car, rushing to be by his side, but got caught in an ice storm. Freezing rain pelted us from all directions. People started using the rocks on the shoulder to move along the roads, just to get a grip. It was as though something was stopping us from getting there on time.

On the way back, I drove. The storm had calmed down, making it easier to manoeuvre on the road. "The Living Years," a song about a man whose father dies before he can say everything he wanted to, came on the radio as we headed home. Suddenly, I felt a tight grip on my arm. I pulled the car to the side of the road, held onto him tight, and we both cried. I cried because he was in pain. I cried because I knew how tough it would be if I were in his situation.

Steve and I broke up over another woman. In the end, it was for the best, because if we hadn't separated, I never would have met Rob.

Rob is where my fantasy world began. And ended.

CHAPTER TWO

Premonitions

As soon as I broke up with Steve, I went out and bought myself a sporty little red RX7 convertible. Even though I knew I would be paying it off for the rest of my life, I didn't care. I wanted to do something for me, something to make me feel good.

The first time I saw Rob was at a bar. There he was, this gorgeous, 6'2" blond muscular man, and I was hooked. I didn't approach him however, because I was too shy. The next day Merk, a patient of mine, came into our office for a cleaning, and I mentioned the man I had seen with him, and how cute I thought he was.

"He said the same thing about you," Merk told me.

"Who is he?!" I asked.

"That's Rob," he told me. "He's single! Want me to set you up?" Silly question.

Rob was in construction, and had been doing renovations on a house down the street from my work. Every lunch hour, I would head over to Cornwall square, and he would watch me walk by in my little white uniform. I had no idea that he had noticed me at all!

Rob took me to Montreal for dinner on our first date. Ten years older than me, Rob had the most beautiful eyes, and a gentle smile. I was hooked instantly. By the end of the evening, he told me he wanted to take me to California. Two weeks later, we went.

California became one of our main vacation spots. We were always going back for one adventure or another. On our first trip we went to Mission Beach, stayed at the Beverly Hills Hotel, toured around Los Angeles, and eventually made our way to San Francisco. On our third trip, we ended up getting licenses to operate 36-foot sailboats. The plan was to sail around the Bay area for two weeks, in preparation for a boating trip to the Virgin Islands. (We never did get there.)

Physical activity was a big deal for Rob, and as a consequence, I found myself becoming more and more active. His goal was to do the Iron Man in Hawaii, and he trained constantly. While he would jog, I would bike along beside him, exhausted by the end of the trip while he had barely broken a sweat. He weighed around 250 lbs., but it was solid muscle. I truly thought I had found Mr. Right. I moved in with him a couple of weeks after our first trip to California. We had only been together a short time, but it felt right.

On my birthday, October 3, 1989, just three months into our relationship, Rob proposed. We were on another trip to California, staying close to Mission Beach. I knew something was up, because all morning he pestered me about the camera case. He kept asking over and over: "Where's the case, Sue? Where's the case?" He was driving me crazy.

"It's right here!" I would tell him over and over.

I was lying on my back, trying to relax in the sun, but Rob kept saying, "Sue? Sue?" over and over, trying to get me to sit up.

"What? The suntan lotion is beside you!"

"Sue? Sue?" Again, he kept trying.

"God, you're being obnoxious today! What is wrong with you?"

Finally I turned towards him. And there he was, holding this little box he'd retrieved from the camera case. His hands were shaking, and big tears had formed in his eyes.

"Oh, my God!" I cried.

Then, I jumped right on top of him. There we were, kissing and rolling around in the sand while the people who walked by tried not to stare. I immediately called my parents to tell them the news. They were happy for me. My father was pleased. The truth was, I had grown distant from my family, especially with my dad. I was so caught up in my life with Rob that I hardly saw them. I was living in my own fantasy world, on a different planet than my parents. I was going on all these exotic trips, and living with this gorgeous man, and I felt like I couldn't relate to them anymore. To this day, I don't know why I felt that way, and I regret that now.

We were planning on eloping to Jamaica. While we had discussed the idea of a traditional wedding, there were too many complications. To begin with, Rob had been married before and he did not have an annulment, which would have been required for a Catholic ceremony. He did talk with a priest about it, but to no avail. So, we ended up with the Jamaica idea. Every time we went away, my family worried I was sneaking off to get married. In the end, we decided against eloping, because too many people would be hurt of we did.

Rob would spoil me with gifts, but my favourite came on Valentine's day. This present was a big, doe-eyed golden Labrador puppy. We named him Mission after our beach, and he went everywhere with us. The cute thing was, we were all blond — an instant family! Mission became my baby, and later on in life, my rock and my true companion.

At this point, we were living in Rob's house on the St. Lawrence River. One evening, in the summertime, as I sat outside watching the sun melt into the water, I started thinking again about how happy I was. My relationship with Rob felt so perfect. And suddenly, I felt a chill run through my body. I get those feelings sometimes, like I know something bad is going to happen. I sensed something foreboding, as much as I didn't want to.

Then, Rob came out to join me. He had just been to a psychic, and the woman had told him that we would help build this beautiful house by the water, that he would get married to a blond that he had met, and there would be a child. She could not see a future for the child, however. The worst thing was, she told him that something bad would happen to him that would set his life back, and that things for him would never be the same after that. We talked about the vision all the time after that.

Rob and I decided to build a home together. We sold his house by the river, and moved into a small apartment where we would live until our A-Frame house had been constructed. It was here, in that cramped space, waiting for our lives to take off in a new direction, that the problems began.

One morning, in the mid-fall of 1991, I was watching the *Today Show* with Katie Couric and Bryant Gumbel as I got ready for work. One of the topics for the day was breast self-examinations. I was still in my bra and underwear, right by the mirror, so I thought I'd try it out.

In my left breast, I found a lump. It was the size of a pea, and it moved around as I touched it. I didn't think much about it, and went back to getting dressed for work.

Later on that night, I got Rob to feel it.

"Yeah, that *is* kind of weird," he agreed. But I changed the topic, not putting too much importance on it.

Over the next couple of weeks, it started to grow; very slightly, but enough to notice. The thing is, once you find something like that in your body, you can't help but touch it constantly. It's like having a loose tooth in your mouth; your tongue always ends up playing with it. Finally, I approached Rob about it again.

"Maybe I should get this checked out," I told him.

"Sure, if you want," he replied. I still wasn't sure, however, so once again, I let it go. But I couldn't get it out of my mind, so I ended up approaching a friend of mine from work, Micheline. I took her to one side, and showed her the lump.

"Touch this," I told her, hesitantly. "Is this normal? Do you think I should worry about it?"

"Get in the back!" she yelled, and I followed her into the back room. "What are you talking about, is this *normal*? I'm calling the doctor *right now*! You aren't getting out of this one!" Within minutes she had booked my appointment. Thrusting the details at me, she again said that I had no choice. I agreed to see the doctor right away.

I parked my car in the back of the clinic and headed inside, convincing myself that this would all be for nothing and that I was fine. Dr. McLean, a large teddy bear of a man, checked out the lump, smiling supportively. I was 24 years old and in good shape, so we were both confident that the lump would turn out to be nothing. It seemed so strange to be in that office.

"As you are young," he told me, "with a firm body, it's probably just a fibroadenoma, which is very common among girls your age. They are just little lumps that come and go." A fibroadenoma is a benign (non-cancerous) tumour which consists of harmless fibrous tissue: little lumps that come and go. But then he added a "however": "We're going to schedule in-and-out surgery," he told me confidently. "We'll have it removed, and you'll be okay. That will be it." While he played down the chances that it actually was a malignant tumour, the sheer fact that the word "cancer" was in our conversation was terrifying.

When I walked out of Dr. McLean's office, I was in a completely different zone. I had no idea where I had parked my car, or what kind of car I was driving; I couldn't even remember if I *had* driven there. Finally, I shook it off, and told myself to get a grip. He said it would be a quick surgery and that I probably had nothing to worry about. The problem was, I had this feeling inside that it wasn't as simple as "in-and-out" surgery, and I couldn't shake it.

My surgery was scheduled for Wednesday, November 27, at the Hôtel Dieu hospital in Cornwall. Even though I had been reassured that I would not be staying overnight, I brought some purple silk pyjamas with me that I had bought with Joanne on one of our shopping excursions. There was no way I was going to be wearing that blue hospital gown. I was prepared, just in case. My mom was with me before I went in, as my father had to work. I sat in a little room, nervously awaiting my turn, trying to think of something else. They administered the anaesthetic, and I drifted off to sleep . . .

I awoke in a room with Dr. McLean at my side. He was all choked up and looked like he had something to tell me. He didn't have to say it; everything was so clear by his pained expression.

I had cancer.

I stared blankly as he explained that they would have to operate again in order to remove the lymph nodes and check if the cancer had spread. Everything was a blur, and I remember the pain that was shared by my loved ones: my mother was crying on the chair. Rob was pacing outside the door, also crying. My father stood by the window, big tears running down his face as his glasses grew misty. As he cried, he prayed: "God, you gave her to us so late in life, why are you coming to take her so quickly?" He came to my bedside and took my hand. Being a religious man he told me and God, right there, that he would quit smoking in order to give me a second chance at life so I could stay here longer with him.

At that point, I had had enough. I bounced out of bed.

"Why is everyone crying so much? I'm not dead yet!"

In the end, I was working at cheering everyone up. The word got around quickly about my diagnosis. My mom phoned the dental clinic, and everyone from work showed up to visit that night: Joanne, Rita, even my boss, Dr. Leboeuf! I felt so loved. Later on, after everyone had left, the weight of the situation hit home. I would be losing 25 percent of my breast as well as some lymph nodes. What if I could never have a child? What if I could never experience that miracle?

The nurses came in, stroking my hand, consoling me as best they could. They told me stories of other women who had made it through just fine.

But at this point, with everyone gone, I couldn't stop crying.

My second surgery was scheduled for Friday. The next day, I found my attitude starting to shift. Dressed in my silk pyjamas, I began putting on my make-up and curling my hair. The nurses kept coming in and laughing kindly at my determined efforts. Rita showed up in mid-preparation, and she also found it amusing.

"I may be dying," I would say, "But I'm going to look good! There are a lot of cute doctors here. Pass me my lipstick!"

I was getting more and more nervous about the following day's surgery — what if the cancer had spread? The fact that I wouldn't get the results until after the weekend was also nerve-wracking. But a new energy started shifting my attitude. Everyone around me kept going on about the importance of thinking positive. So, I decided that it was time to take control.

Rob had bought me a CD walkman to listen to in the hospital. Before they took me to surgery, I made sure to put my Bob Marley CD inside. I advanced to the song "Three Little Birds," the song I had been listening to over and over:

"Don't worry, 'bout a thing . . . 'cause every little thing's gonna be all right."

I didn't want the doctors treating me like just another number. I wanted them to know that I was Suzanne Giroux, and I was special. I wanted them to remember me. So, as I lay there, surrounded by a sea of green gowns, flip-flops, hats, and masks, I made a decision. I sat up, one earphone in my ear, and the other in my hand and I thrust it toward one of the surgeons.

"Here! Put this in your ear!"

The first surgeon listened to Bob Marley croon away, a smile on his face. One by one, I made them all listen to a piece of the song. Finally, one of the nurses put the earphone back in my ear. They all laughed, reassuring me.

"Don't worry! Don't worry!"

My family doctor, Dr. Agatha Forson, was the one putting me under, which was reassuring. So I lay back down, with Bob telling me once again that everything was going to be all right, and I fell asleep.

According to my medical files, I had an axillary node dissection done on my left breast, along with the removal of a gland from the left axilla. In other words, they took out some of the lymph nodes from under my arm, and also took out a gland. The "tissue removed" — my breast — is described as follows: "two-thirds are greyish-brown, slightly indurated [hard] and one-third is bright yellow, soft, and fatty."

The results came back negative, which was a huge relief. The next step was radiation therapy, which I would undergo for five weeks at Ottawa General Hospital. I would stay in a special wing set up for cancer patients undergoing treatment during the week, then come home to Rob and my family on the weekends.

The hospital staff had tried to set up the room assignments to match personalities, and my roommate, Ghislaine Gregoire, turned out to be fantastic. She was around 40 years old, very cool, spunky, and friendly. We would go to our five-minute treatments, then after that we'd go shopping, grab some lunch, and hang out, wandering around Ottawa. It was just like being on holiday! We spent so much time together because the majority of the people in the ward were too sick to go out. At nights, in the lounge, we would take over the karaoke machine, and I would sing to the other cancer patients. I certainly wasn't brilliant, but I had a few Karen Carpenter songs that I liked to do and it was fun. The porters found out about it, and kept asking to let them know when I'd be singing next so they could catch the show! It was winter, and as we were there for five weeks it was the only way we could entertain ourselves.

The radiation treatments themselves were quick. The first thing they did was make a plaster mould of my upper body. Next, I was pinned to a table with my arms placed above my head under a plastic shield that was made from the mould. Then, they would draw little lines over the shield, indicating the precise area that needed to be treated with radiation. The doctors would leave the room, and a large machine would be placed over my chest. It was definitely a scary experience. I kept staring at this big machine wondering what it would feel like.

"You won't feel anything," the staff reassured me. And I didn't. I just stared up at the ceiling, losing myself in pictures of scenery that had been stuck up there. And *zap* . . . for five minutes. That was it.

After the first time, the treatments were easy because I knew what to expect. I used to joke with the technicians after they bolted me down: "Hey! If there's a fire, you guys aren't forgetting me here!" Joking somehow made it easier. My left breast was growing firmer due to the radiation, so with every check-up I'd make sure to joke with the doctor about giving me a quick buzz on the other side as well! (Just to keep things even, you know . . .) Otherwise, I was quite lucky when it came to physical side effects. I had a mild burn from the treatment, but not half as bad as some of the other women there. There were a few that had raw, blistered breasts after the first week. Radiation is like having a sunburn over a sunburn, and you know the treatments aren't going to stop.

None of my family came to see me in Ottawa while I was on treatment, but that was because I gave them all the impression that the treatments were not a big deal. I never asked them to come up and see me. It helped that I had such great support from my roommate, and I was going home each weekend. As soon as I got home, I would be all over Rob, starved for physical affection. Then, tough as it was, I would head back for my next week of treatment.

And then, I got pregnant.

My period was late. At first I didn't think anything of it, but in the end, I did the test and sure enough, it was positive. I had to talk to a specialist to see if I could even keep the child after it had been exposed to so much radiation. They did all sorts of tests, the main question being whether or not the baby was normal after such exposure. I was terrified at the idea of my child having a birth defect, and my relationship with Rob was going through a lot of strain as it was. I knew he didn't want to be in that situation, not when we had only one household income and I was still undergoing treatment for cancer. How could I blame him?

The doctors warned me that if the radiation exposure had been too great, the baby would die. My heart was breaking, but I had no choice. Abortion was the only real solution. I had to make my final decision the day they did the ultrasound. But when I got there, the doctor informed me that the baby had already died in the womb. I couldn't understand — I hadn't bled, or anything that I could remember. It had only been three months old. The doctors continued on with the D & C, and I was left to deal with the pain — both physical and emotional.

Near the end of the five weeks, I was so homesick and I missed Rob so much, I made the decision to make the daily trip to Ottawa from home. It was only an hour's drive there and back, but people kept telling me I would be too drained and sleepy from the treatment to do it. I did it anyway, and felt tired only at the very end of the treatment. Once I was back at home for good, I had to rest and let my immune system build itself up again. A nurse came to our place for a week to clean my burn, drain the area, and change the dressing.

At the time, I didn't know about detoxifying my system or changing my diet to help my body heal. I saw it as an episode in life that I got through, then life went on. As far as I was concerned, I was 24 years old, and certainly had no risk of dying. I was completely living in a world of my own, not facing the reality. Today I see children dying of cancer all the time, but then, I was blind to the seriousness of the situation. I was convinced it wasn't my time and that was that.

At the end of my radiation treatments, we moved into the A-frame house. Once I was healthy again, I went to Dr. Luc Leboeuf in the hopes that I could get my job back. Unfortunately, he wasn't in a position to hire me back straight away, so I was unemployed. I still had major car payments that I couldn't afford, and Rob was also having money troubles. Tensions started to pop up between us, and things were rocky for a while. The topic of marriage wasn't discussed for some time.

Life continued, and time healed a few wounds. Once again, Rob and I were back in love. I had become more reflective about things, however. I shared with Rob that I had a feeling I would never have children, even though a family of my own was what I wanted most. Looking back, it was something I always believed, even when I was a child myself. It made me start to question just what my destiny was.

The wedding plans came into effect. Rob and I invited our priest over one Saturday night for a pow-wow session with my parents, as well as a nice dinner. That night, I made love to him, and I found myself crying. I had the strangest feeling he was slipping away from me. The next day, Sunday, he got out of bed to do some quick work on his job site.

"No," I pleaded. "Don't go. It's Sunday. You're not supposed to work on Sunday."

"I'm just going until noon," he reassured me. "Then I'll be back."

Rob left, and I still felt uncomfortable. I sat on the couch, debating over and over in my head whether or not I should take a shower. I decided not to. Just then, the telephone rang.

"Sue?" It was the man whose house Rob was working on. "Rob had an accident. He's on his way to the hospital . . . I think you should be there."

Suddenly I remembered what the psychic had said to him: *"Something bad will happen that will set your life back . . ."*

"Oh my God . . ." I thought, as I pulled myself together. I got dressed as fast as I could and raced to the car. The closer I got to the hospital, the stronger the feeling got; he was disconnecting from me. I burst into the ER, and when I saw him, I knew how serious it was. He had fallen on his head and was suffering from major brain damage, and he hadn't said a word since the fall. I moved closer, and he spoke.

"Baby, is that you?"

The nurses and doctors went nuts as soon as he opened his mouth, panicking about internal swelling and pressure on the brain. They injected him with something, knocking him out. Those were his last words to me.

His last words.

They flew him to Ottawa straight away. I was falling into a personal hell and couldn't even think straight because it was all happening so quickly. My whole family and I followed behind. It was one of the hardest times in my life. Rob's parents soon arrived, along with Merk, who had introduced us so long ago. When we got there, they put us in a little room. It's always a little room when the news is bad. The doctors told us more surgery was required to remove more brain tissue. His brain was so badly damaged that they couldn't keep the swelling down. It was a nightmare.

No one knew how he had fallen on his head. He had been building a house, but the stairs hadn't been put in yet. There was speculation that he had had an aneurysm first, causing him to fall. Otherwise, it didn't make sense. He was tall and strong and he could have grabbed something. How could he have fallen on his head? The doctors never found out, and it remains a mystery.

After Rob's accident, my parents took me back to their house. A good friend of mine called up, telling me about her recent engagement, and I couldn't handle it. I had just lost that dream. I ran a bath, and then I broke down completely. My mother came in, holding me tightly, unsure of what to do. My father was dealing with phone calls from concerned friends, while my mother did her best to console me. Finally, they got me dressed and took me to the hospital where Dr. Forson gave me a sedative.

Eventually, because I was his fiancée, I had to sign the release papers along with his mother allowing Rob to die. It was one of the hardest choices I had to make. That night, exhausted, in the Journey's Inn with my family, I cried for hours on end believing he was gone. The next morning, however, the hospital called us up to let us know that Rob had made it through the night. He was still alive. They had known hours earlier, but they hadn't called because they thought I needed some rest. So, back we went — back to reconcile ourselves with his condition once more.

Rob had a stroke after that. He underwent so many different surgeries, I lost count. In the end, half of his left frontal lobe was removed. The whole situation lasted about a year. He remained in the hospital for a long, long time. Eventually, he was moved to a home where they could take better care of him. He is still there today and can function now, but the man I knew is gone.

During the time he was in the hospital, I started having difficulties with his parents. His mother wanted me to see a lawyer, as she wanted to start dividing up our property. While she tried to take control of the situation, I tried to deal with my grief. I couldn't even comprehend the idea. All I was trying to do was be by his bedside. I had no interest in lawyers. They were even trying to take Mission, but I wouldn't have it. It was yet another situation that was draining the life out of me. I was reaching a breaking point.

Christmas came. My emotions were running high, and I was hurting terribly. I had started working at a restaurant to make some money. One night I was approached by a woman who claimed to have had an affair with Rob while we had been together. It was the straw that broke the camel's back, or in this case, mine. Feeling betrayed, and frustrated at being unable to communicate with Rob, I went off to a Christmas party and got extremely drunk. In that state, I stupidly decided to get into my car and drive to Ottawa to confront him.

At the hospital, upon seeing him, I broke down once more, flooded with emotion. I sat down by his bed, and over and over asked him "Why? Why?" as I cried uncontrollably. A blank look rested on his face. I knew he couldn't answer. Finally, a nurse saw me, and took me into another room. She counselled me as best she could, trying to calm me down. I finally fell asleep. The next morning, I woke up and left.

It was the last time I went to the hospital.

Driving home that morning, I ran out of gas about 500 feet from a station. A cop filling up there helped me push my car right up to the pumps. Between running out of gas right by a station, and safely making it to Ottawa when I was in no state to drive, I knew that someone must have been looking out for me, and for that, I was grateful.

Rob and I were together for three and a half years. And then, in one instant, it was over. I was left in debt, with an empty house full of broken dreams.

The road ahead was dark . . . and I had a long way to go.

CHAPTER THREE

Little Girl Lost

After Rob's accident, my whole life turned upside down. For a brief time, I moved back in with my parents, simply because I was too afraid to be alone, and I couldn't handle seeing all of Rob's things. After a month, however, I had to return to the A-frame house Rob and I had just moved into, and deal with reality. Jobless and emotionally drained, I had to find the will to keep on living.

I was right behind the eight ball financially. Suddenly, there were all these payments that I had never noticed before: electricity, cable, hydro . . . not to mention my car and house payments! I had always let Rob do everything for me, so I never knew what sort of money we owed. When the time came to pay, I had no idea where to start.

I was desperate. So I came up with an idea.

I knew Rob had a connection to a guy working as a smuggler. About a week before his accident, Rob had mentioned this man, and how much money he was making. It was common in those days in Cornwall to smuggle cigarettes into Quebec. The cigarettes would come up from the U.S. via the Native Americans on the island across from Cornwall. Because the taxes on cigarettes were so high at that time, the smugglers were making huge amounts of money. So I decided to call the man up, and see if I could meet with him. He agreed, and I showed up at his home one Sunday after he had returned from church. I presented my situation, and asked if I could do some work for him — anything — because I needed it desperately. He offered, and I accepted.

I started smuggling. All I had to do was drive a pickup truck filled with boxes to Montreal, then back it up to the loading dock and sit in the truck until it was unloaded. Once it was empty, I would return to Cornwall to pick up my payment. That first time, I made a high three figure number for an hour's drive. More money than I'd ever made in a day! Some days, I made triple that amount. *Triple!*

It was during this period of my life that I met my best friend, Jodi Lyn Hawkshaw, through mutual friends. With short dark hair and large mischievous eyes, Jodi Lyn is like a sister to me. We would fight like cats and dogs, then two minutes later, everything would be forgotten. She not only helped keep me sane, but she helped me to move on as well. Gone was the bleached blond hair, blue eyeliner, and pink lipstick. Suddenly, I had rich, auburn hair and a subtler look. We would giggle over everything, talking late into the night about men, life, and her dream to become a professional country singer. My dreams had vanished so fast, I didn't know what to dream about anymore, so I enjoyed listening to hers.

I was living in an empty house, and feeling extremely lonely, so Jodi Lyn moved in with me. She was a lifesaver. Seeing as the house was open concept, the master bedroom had no doors; it just sat on a second-level balcony that overlooked the living room. For the first few nights, Jodi Lyn and I would talk back and forth as she lay in bed downstairs. Eventually, she would climb up and join me, neither of us wanting to be alone.

During the smuggling I was still in court with Rob's parents. They wanted the house and my dog Mission, and they fought me for it. Suddenly, I was paying for court fees as well. In the end, the judge sympathized with me, claiming that the whole situation had been a waste of the court's time and that I had been through enough. Rob's parents took his things, and I was required to move once more, but Mission stayed with me. I was so lost in my own world that the whole situation became a blur.

My other friends were starting to sense that something was up. When I went up to visit with my friend Rita in Montreal, all she knew was that I had no job, was in debt, and was still struggling with losing Rob. She had planned on buying me a nice meal, knowing I had very little money. Imagine her surprise when the first thing I suggested we do was go shopping! There I was, going into different stores and shelling out money for different expensive items, with Rita staring at me oddly. I kept my secret to myself.

I would offer to lend money to different friends and bought lots of new furniture, racing around in my red car. My friends knew I could be a risk taker, and their concern for my welfare was evident. I was living the high life, however, not letting myself see the danger of what I was doing. It wasn't just Rob I lost after the accident, but my dream of a fairy-tale life. I was able to deal with the cancer because I had had him by my side. With him gone, I avoided reality for fear of falling apart.

Jodi Lyn and I took spontaneity to a new level. We would head off on different adventures in my little RX7. We'd just hop in and take off wherever we felt like. Often, we'd head to Toronto or Montreal. One time, we packed up the car with both our winter and summer clothing, planning on heading to Atlantic City to win some money first, then head down to Florida. (We never made it far, though.) Wherever we went, we'd have sore stomachs from laughing, and we'd always end up coming home.

At this point, I met up with a man called Paul in a local bar. He was in town drawing cartoon maps of Cornwall and was tall, dark, and handsome. I started telling him about Rob, and the attraction between us blossomed. He was in town temporarily, but while he was there, we grew close. There were many nights where he would console me, staying by my side as I would fall asleep crying over Rob. He moved back to Toronto, making my trips there more frequent. He was a very good friend.

Going to Toronto to visit Paul allowed me to escape everything I couldn't face in Cornwall. Depression continued to lurk inside me. I turned away from my whole family, hardly speaking to them and rarely visiting. For a year, it was like I fell off the face of the earth and I focused on smuggling and spending the money. My father knew something was seriously wrong right from the start. He tried to get the truth out of me, but I just couldn't bear to tell him. I was ashamed about what I was doing, and he could read me like a book. So, I kept my distance, spending all my time at bars, at restaurants, throwing away money foolishly, and drinking. I was lost, with no idea how to get back on track.

Then, I got caught.

I was driving my biggest load, 60 boxes. Someone had snitched on me. Suddenly, there I was, confronted by the police and facing an immense fine. The shame I felt before was nothing compared to how I felt now. That was the end of my party days. I lost my little red car because I had foolishly declined to buy insurance, and I couldn't afford the car payments anymore. I had to move to a smaller place. I declared personal bankruptcy. When things got dark and scary for me, my first reaction was to leave: to do something drastic. But I didn't have the strength. There was nothing I could do but keep going.

But things never stay normal for long.

Paul and I were still seeing each other, but the long distance relationship was difficult for me. My friend Lynn from high school was seeing Stephane, my grade 10 crush. His hair was shorter and dark, a change from the blond curls in high school. The four of us started getting together whenever Paul came up to visit me. Not long afterwards, I began visiting with them myself. Soon, I was going over frequently for suppers. There were occasions where Steph and I would flirt harmlessly, but it was nothing serious. Then, one morning, suffering a little from a night of partying, I dropped by their place for a visit. Lynn was showing me the large containers of food she had gotten from the Price Club, and I mentioned how I would love to go some time. Steph mentioned that he was making a trip there the following day.

"Lynn, you don't mind if she joins me?" Steph asked.

Of course, she didn't mind at all.

After we hit the Price Club, Steph and I took a drive through Rosemont, a wealthier suburb of Montreal. Seeing all these beautiful homes, then heading out for an elegant lunch filled with wine and a fine variety of fruit and cheese was so decadent, but wonderful. Extravagance was something I had always wanted. I loved beautiful things, and he knew it. The nice thing was, he loved them too. Even though I was with Paul, I still felt at the end of my rope. Steph made me feel as though I was being taken care of; it was exactly what I was craving.

Not too long afterwards, I had to move again, this time to an even smaller apartment. Money was tight, and I couldn't afford my place anymore. Steph volunteered to help me move. As I lugged the boxes outside, a knife fell from one, cutting my foot. I reached down to check it out, when suddenly Steph was right beside me, picking up the knife.

And he kissed me.

I stood up, telling him he shouldn't be doing that. I felt terrible. And yet, I was attracted to him.

The next day, he showed up at my new apartment.

"What are you doing here?" I questioned him.

"Well," he said, "I thought something happened."

"Oh, no," I told him weakly. "No."

But it had.

Lynn, Steph, Paul, and I had planned a weekend together down at the Skydome in Toronto. We would all meet up, watch a baseball game, and stay overnight in the hotel. But now Steph and I had kissed, and things were different. The fact was, Paul was in Toronto, while Steph was in Cornwall. I needed to be with someone who could be there for me. I explained the situation to Paul and it was an amicable breakup. That night, Steph drove Lynn back to Cornwall and broke it off with her. It wasn't a situation that I was proud of. It just happened.

Six weeks later, I moved in with him.

At the beginning of our relationship, he was constantly with me. He owned a business in town, but for those first weeks he avoided his office and did all his work through his cell phone. We would go out for picnics, and he would lavish me with flowers and dinners. Our relationship was filled with extravagance.

The first time my parents met Steph, my mother recognized his name. She asked Steph who his father was, only to discover it was Pierre, the man who had counselled her years before. Even though they were uncomfortable with the situation, my parents made an effort when it came to gatherings with Steph's family.

Jodi Lyn would come over and keep me company whenever Steph was away for work reasons. We would laugh, enjoy some wine, and take turns cooking meals. And then, one night, while I was asleep at home, Jodi Lyn ran into Steph at a bar. The next day, she called to talk, telling me Steph had made a pass at her. I refused to listen to her story and told her she was wrong. Hanging up the phone, I pushed down the pain. After that incident, Steph no longer seemed to like Jodi Lyn, so I stayed away from her in order to avoid arguments. My closest friend, and I cut her off because I couldn't face the brutal truth: my relationship was not as ideal as it had seemed.

Pushing doubts aside, things with Steph continued to be filled with romance. One day, Steph and I made up a special picnic and found a lovely, secluded spot by a beach. He had pulled out his laptop, and we started playing on it as we sipped wine. It was there, in this unique setting, that I had one of my inklings. Steph had decided he wanted to marry me. I knew it in my heart. For years we looked for that same spot, but we never found it again.

Not too long afterwards, we planned a large dinner for our families. Steph had intended to propose to me, then announce it at dinner. I had just drawn a bath, and was soaking quietly by myself, when he appeared at the door with a bouquet of roses. Excitedly, he presented them to me, waiting expectantly. I leaned over to admire them.

Inside was a diamond ring.

Steph had been married before, with a son from his previous marriage, but I believed we could make it work. I thought, finally, I could have the dream I'd dreamt for so long: the white picket fence. The children running around with their father. To be a happy family.

And yet, I knew something was wrong.

With Rob, everything felt right. With Steph, I had my concerns. Our engagement lasted a year before we had the wedding. Not only that, but his previous marriage had not ended well. Finally, we set the date: September 30, 1994, just three days before my twenty-seventh birthday. I decided to move out of the house a week before the wedding so our wedding night would be more special. My cousin, Manon, had just had a little boy, and invited me to live with her for the time being. I heard later Steph had a good time with his friends that week. The problem was, we both had our reservations about the wedding, which was not a good start.

It was an extremely hectic time, and I was stressing out. I was paranoid that Steph would stand me up on the wedding day. Steph wanted to avoid inviting some of his closer relatives, so that meant I couldn't invite mine. That was a tough decision, considering how close I was to my aunt and uncle. It was to be my parents, his father and sister, and a few friends. My cousins showed up to the ceremony regardless, but they were terribly hurt at being excluded. I didn't blame them one bit.

The ceremony was at a Catholic church, with Rita, my closest friend since my fight with Jodi Lyn, as my maid of honour. Both my parents walked me down the aisle. My long hair was swept up, with a few ringlets hanging down. My white gown was floor length, with long sleeves, and puffed shoulders. The final touch was a delicate tiara nestled in my hair. White flowered embroidery decorated the hem of the dress, as well as the open neckline, and I carried red roses as my bouquet. Steph looked elegant in his classic tuxedo, his dark hair neatly combed back. My nervousness started to fade.

The reception was held at an old manor called the Georgian House. The menu offered a selection of delights from prime rib to lobster tail. I allowed myself to relax, thinking of my upcoming honeymoon. We had planned to stay at his father's cottage in the Laurentians for a few days, then head down to New York City to visit with his sister. The whole honeymoon would last for a week.

But things started to fall apart right from the start.

That first night, after arriving at the cottage, Steph approached me on a rather delicate matter. Steph told me of a girl named Carole, who was going through a rough time, and he asked me if I minded helping her out. This girl wanted to be a pharmaceutical technician, but in order for her to do so, she needed to take a specific course. The problem was, she had no money, and her father was sick, and so forth. Apparently, she had no one to help her, and Steph suggested that we give her some money each month to get by.

I couldn't believe it. It was my wedding night and here was my husband asking me if we could support another woman! I flipped out. We started arguing quite heavily that night.

I let it go, and Steph apologized the next day. We spent the rest of the time at the cottage boating, then headed down to New York to see his sister, France. We did the usual sightseeing while we were there, checking out all that New York had to offer. It was enjoyable, but we rushed back to Cornwall as Steph informed me that he had a lot of work to catch up on. The honeymoon was over, and as I was not working, I got into the housewife role.

That first day back in Cornwall, Steph phoned me up, saying he had to head up to Kingsy Falls in northern Quebec for a meeting. He asked me if I would pack him a bag, and iron his beige pants and red shirt. I agreed, but as I hung up the phone, I knew something was wrong. He took off, but didn't call me that night. By the time he returned to town, it was the weekend.

His young son, Alex, was in town visiting us. Some Sundays when Alex came to see us, Steph would take him to his friend Stefan's home to play with Stef's kids while he and Stef went to watch Formula One racing. While they were out, I started cleaning up Steph's office, and I stumbled upon a receipt. Assuming it was from his meeting, I took a look at it.

It was for a Best Western Hotel in Montreal.

I checked the dates. They matched the ones from the past week. He had not been in Kingsy Falls at all. I headed straight for the phone, and called up Stefan's wife, Cathy. She told me not to panic, that there may be a logical explanation. After hanging up the phone, I calmed down a bit. Still, I wasn't convinced. I returned to the office, searching for any other incriminating evidence.

I found it.

It was a receipt for $298 dollars spent at a store in Montreal called Boutique de Seduction. I headed straight for the phone once more.

"Oh, boy . . ." Cathy said. "Why don't you come on over, we'll have a coffee, and you can relax. We'll take care of Alex, and you can talk to Steph when he gets here."

My heart was racing, and my emotions high. I felt angry and betrayed, not wanting to believe that my suspicions were correct.

Steph and Stefan turned up the drive. I waited outside while Cathy stood at the door. He saw my car, then me.

"What are you doing?"

"Get in the car," I told him coldly, meaning mine.

"Well, Alex —" he started.

"— it's okay," Cathy said. "I think you guys need to talk."

"What's going on? What's going on?" he kept asking.

"Get in the car," I repeated, struggling to keep from crying.

Alex continued to play with Cathy's boys, and Steph and I got inside my car.

I confronted him about the Best Western receipt.

"Oh, well, yeah," he said, "I came back to town and we had the meeting in Montreal instead —" Then, he turned on me, "What were you doing snooping in the first place?"

"I'm not done with you!" I shouted. "Did you buy your friend some Boutique de Seduction? What the hell is that all about? I know you probably went to see Carole!"

He admitted to me that he had seen Carole, but he had done so in order to tell her it was over.

"So you take her shopping to Boutique de Seduction to buy her *$298 worth of stuff?!* And then spend the night at the Best Western on Crescent?! What do you think I am, stupid?! Why couldn't you just do it over the phone? *We just got back from our honeymoon!*"

Well, that was a total disaster. I burst into tears, crying over and over. Poor Alex ended up at Cathy's while we argued until eight o'clock at night. Finally, we drove home and I went to bed.

I couldn't erase the thought of Steph with another woman from my mind, even though he claimed nothing had happened with Carole. There were nights he went out drinking with friends and came home late, and every time he walked out that door my trust was tested, and my self-esteem grew lower and lower.

I didn't want to see the truth. I had created a very specific image of Steph in my mind. That Steph was the loving husband I had always wanted. He was the man who spoiled me rotten, buying me beautiful flowers and clothing, taking me out for wonderful suppers after long days of work. That Steph took wacky pictures with me and Alex when he came to visit, and took me on vacations. The arguments and the late nights away from home kept being pushed to one side, even though it was eating me up. I wanted this marriage to work, and I was going to do everything I could in order to do so.

I returned to work for Dr. Leboeuf not too long after our honeymoon. Soon, Steph and I had fallen into a nice daily routine. He was the early bird, heading off to work at 6 a.m., while I would sleep in for a bit. Once Steph drove off, Mission would jump up into the bed and cuddle with me. Steph did not like Mission sleeping in the bed, so we had to keep it our secret. We would cuddle for a short time, then I would get up and dress for work. Steph would call me there around midday to see how my day had gone. If it had been a tough day, he would take me out to dinner that night. Otherwise, I would head home and prepare supper.

Then, there were the nights where I fell asleep on the couch as I watched movies, wondering where he was and when he would come home. The ache in my stomach became constant. Having good friends to talk to kept me sane, yet while they were there for me, there are still those moments when you are alone and have to face the world by yourself. I kept focusing on the good times. But while there were good times with Steph, there were also a mounting number of problems.

I thought things would change when we decided to do renovations on our small, three bedroom house. The plan was to redo the entire kitchen and break a couple of walls down, opening up the main floor.

We also wanted a new bathroom in the basement, with a large jacuzzi-style bathtub. The whole process would cost around $50,000 and last for approximately six months. For the duration, we planned to live in a friend's cottage in Lancaster. Steph and I had been married for about a year at this point, and I still believed we had a chance. Moving into the beautiful A-frame cottage with a large stone fireplace right by the water meant moving out of the city. My thinking was, if we were away from the city there would be fewer nights where Steph was away from home. That was what I was hoping, anyway.

Living in Lancaster had its moments. We moved in during the summer, which was lovely. My father and mother would come up and visit me frequently, spending time just hanging out. We would go out fishing off the dock. When Alex came to visit, we would go camping, or canoe and swim around the lake. We'd have to put Mission in the canoe with us, because we couldn't leave him alone on the dock. Every time we tried, he would jump in the water, swimming furiously after us. Then, there were the lazy days where we would just relax, and hang out with friends. There'd be the occasional splash in the background as Mission dived in the water, chasing after the fish. The theme was "fun fun fun."

But things weren't as perfect as they seemed. The fact was, Steph still had many late nights away from home. The television only offered a few old programs, taking away one distraction I craved on lonely nights. Being alone in the house was scarier because it was two miles from the main road, and as the seasons changed, it grew darker earlier each night. Some mornings, as late as 5 a.m., I would wake up alone to the sound of Steph's truck coming down the road. And yet, the next day, we would fall into the same routine all over again. It was as though nothing had happened.

I had turned to our friends Paul and Jody Marleau at this point. Jody was a social worker, someone with whom I could talk candidly. And yet, while I knew there were problems, I still didn't want to face them head on. They came to visit us one time, knowing full well what the situation was. A vase filled with roses from Steph was sitting on one of the tables, and Paul asked why they were there, hoping it was for a good reason. I had learned very quickly how to look as though nothing was wrong, but I felt as though Paul could see through the façade.

We returned to our newly renovated home in October, and things kept going on just as they always had. Steph seemed wonderful one moment, and cruel the next. My family knew there were problems, but I didn't want to face them, so they didn't force me. The fact was, we put on a good show. And the happy moments *did* continue throughout. We had dinners out with friends, keeping ourselves socially active. We would sit and talk as he took his bath. For his thirtieth birthday, I arranged for a surprise party with all his close friends and family present. I had fooled him completely, casually brushing off our dinner plans for the evening. He got there and was thrilled. It was a lovely evening. It was in those moments that I found myself believing that things would be different.

Then, we decided to try and have a child. It was a chance for us, and I wanted so much to have a family, so in April 1997, I got pregnant. I was a hormonal basket case. I couldn't stop throwing up, and was moody and weepy all the time. Despite it all, I was happy. I started shopping for my unborn daughter early, excited for her arrival. I had decided on the name Shanelle, because I wanted it to match Suzanne and Stephane. I wanted her so much, and yet I was always terrified of losing her.

So, three months later, in June, when I started bleeding, I desperately tried not to think the worst. The doctors did an amniocentesis test through my belly button to determine what was going on. The results came in, and they informed me that my baby had died inside of my womb. Three months old.

I woke up after they had finished the D & C, and I couldn't quite grasp that my baby was gone. I knew this was my last chance to have a child, and I had lost her. I couldn't talk to people about it; I didn't want to. Instead, I returned home and gave Shanelle's stuff to my sister-in-law and a couple of other friends. Steph kept his pain to himself.

On Father's Day, I took my parents to Mt. Tremblant. It was a Sunday, and Steph opted to go watch Formula One racing. I didn't mind, as it was a chance for my parents and I to spend time together alone. We sat out at a café, sipping red wine, enjoying the sunshine. Later, we went for a ride on the chair lift. As we headed up, Dad would smile at the people heading down. Finally, he threw his arm around me, pretending I was his "young" girlfriend. Giddy from wine and laughter, we finally reached the top. The view was spectacular. It was a beautiful moment, a perfect moment. And yet, somewhere deep inside of me, all the way up the mountain, I knew in my soul that something bad was going to happen, just as I had felt it with Rob.

Yet, so many bad things *had* happened, and I couldn't bear to contemplate any more. Instead, I took my father's arm, pushed all thoughts out of my mind, and enjoyed the rest of our day together.

CHAPTER FOUR

Death ... and Rebirth

The summer had come to a close, and we had just started another September. Once again, Steph and I had slipped back into routine. Princess Diana had just been killed in a major car accident, and Mother Teresa's death followed that same weekend. I was a great admirer of both women, and was completely shocked and upset at the loss. Due to the time difference with London, Princess Diana's funeral had been quite early in the morning. I made sure to record it, planning on watching it later.

I went to work that morning with a sore throat. I continued working, but soon I was feeling short of breath. Finally, I asked Dr. LeBoeuf if it was all right for me to head over to the Hôtel Dieu hospital during my lunch break in order to get some antibiotics. I figured I must have the flu, or something, but I really wasn't sure. When I got there, the doctors gave me a chest X-ray, diagnosing me with pneumonia. They told me to go home and get some rest. I went back to work first, and finished my day there. But it was starting to get worse as the day continued.

That night, I could hardly breathe, especially when I tried lying down on my back. Not only that, but my stomach had started to swell. So, Steph took me to the hospital again. We waited for two hours, only to be told that the antibiotics hadn't affected my system yet. They prescribed me stronger ones and sent me home. I knew there must be more to it, however, because of my stomach bloating. Instead of arguing the matter, we headed back home. Somehow, I managed to fall asleep.

The next morning, I looked eight months pregnant. I sat down with Steph and asked him what I should do.

"Ah, you'll be fine," he reassured me. But I could see the concern in his eyes.

I tried to let it go, because I figured the doctors must know what they were talking about, but a sneaking thought remained in the back of my head. Trying to distract myself, I sat down and started watching Princess Diana's funeral. I watched as different people spoke about her, this woman whom I respected, who had done such admirable work. I kept thinking, this shows you how precious life is, when anyone can go just like that.

On that thought, I made a decision. I picked up the phone and called up my family doctor, Dr. Forson. She had been there during my cancer and when Rob's accident occurred. I didn't expect to get a hold of her — she was so busy all the time, it was almost impossible to track her down. And yet, when I called that day, not only was she in her office, but she answered the phone personally. As far as I was concerned, that was a sign.

"Get over to the hospital," she told me. "I'm going to go in and check you out. I was actually on my way there." I headed over straight away, and Dr. Forson examined me. Upon first examination, she directed me immediately to Dr. Dennis Pyne, a surgeon at the hospital. Right after, they started doing a whole series of different tests on me. The bloating was worse, and I found I couldn't even manage to breathe anymore. Suddenly, I was vomiting fluid as it continued to build up inside of me. They tried an ultrasound, but found nothing. The problem was, no one had any idea what was going on. As I fell in and out of consciousness, I remember lying in a room with a nurse who was attempting to get my blood pressure. The problem was, she couldn't find my second pulse. Suddenly, another nurse came. And another. And another. Within moments, I heard Dr. Pyne being paged over the intercom to come quickly. Then, I slipped out of consciousness.

Moments later, I was awake again. Now the doctors wanted to fly me to Ottawa. The problem was they had no time, and my body wouldn't have been able to stand the pressure up in a helicopter. Driving me there was also out of the question. I didn't have an hour to spare at this point. Everything around me was getting more and more hectic. I was so frightened, simply because I didn't know what the hell was going on. I could hear my father out in the hallway, desperately yelling for someone to do something. *Anything.*

My father was always my voice when I couldn't speak. Lying there, half-conscious, Dad became my eyes, my voice, and my guardian. Monitors were beeping all around me, giving me frightening flashbacks of Rob. That sharp sound reminded me of what happened to him, along with that distinctive smell that only hospitals have. It scared the hell out of me.

And yet, even though everything around me was so hectic and dramatic, somewhere inside myself I knew it wasn't my time. It was a Saturday night, and my whole family was with me. No one was sure whether or not I was going to make it. The priest arrived to perform the last rites while my family kept by my side, telling me to hang in there. There I was, watching everybody weeping and all I could think was, I'm going to get out of this one, too.

So, with no other options left, the doctors performed exploratory surgery in the hopes that they would not only save me, but would figure out what was going on.

Dr. Pyne managed to save me, and yet they still had no clue what was causing the buildup of fluid. Not only was it in my lungs and liver, but it was surrounding my heart, cutting off its ability to pump blood. If we had waited any longer, I would have gone into cardiac arrest. Dr. Pyne tested for a whole plethora of illnesses that I hadn't even heard of, including flesh-eating diseases and exotic viruses. They scheduled a second surgical operation for me, still unsure what they were looking for.

My family stood by me, telling me over and over again to "think positive." I felt like saying "Why don't you step into my shoes and see if you can think positive?" I know everyone does their best to cope in a situation like that, trying to come to terms with what is happening, but I began to wonder what it was they thought I was thinking. "Think positive? Hell, no. I'm just feeling sorry for myself, and hopefully I'll croak." Hey, I want to stick around, too! I'm doing what I can. It's a hard thing, to think you are going to die. You can see the pain in the people's faces around you, and you want so much to reassure them. The irony is, that's what they are trying to do for you.

Having the priest there repeatedly performing last rites wasn't exactly helping my morale, either. I now had six tubes the size of small hoses coming out of my body, draining the fluid as it continued to build: two on each side, and two below me. In addition to those, I was hooked up to a catheter to drain my urine, an IV to replenish my fluids, and God knows how many monitors around me. I looked like an octopus.

Because they weren't sure if I would survive the operation, the doctor asked if there was any last thing I would like to happen before I went into surgery.

"I want to see Mission," I told him.

Bringing a dog into the hospital had never happened before. Steph, however, had a connection through one of the hospital directors. Both of them cycled together at the Cornwall Cycling Club. Steph told him my situation and how difficult it was for him, and how much I wanted to see my dog. The director showed a lot of compassion, and allowed it. Suddenly, Mission was there, at the doorway. When he saw me, he jumped right on my bed. It was painful, considering all the tubes I had coming out of me, but I didn't care. Steph looked so lost, watching Mission and I. The nurses burst into tears at the scene, while my family and friends kept repeating: "You're going to make it. You're strong. Don't worry."

I prayed right then: "Please, God. Give me a second chance. The first time you gave it to me, but I did nothing with it. This time I'll find a purpose. I'll work at helping people see hope in their situations. Please."

I felt like I had done nothing with my life, or made a difference. I wanted Suzanne Giroux to be someone who had an impact on others. Who *did* something. I prayed that God would grant me that opportunity.

The doctors didn't think I would survive the second operation. My father was devastated, while my mother was exhausted and emotionally tortured. There I was, their only child, with all these tubes coming out of her, hooked up to so many machines with no idea if I would make it from one moment to the next. Finally, they wheeled me away.

And I made it. After surgery, I was readmitted to the intensive care unit. At that point, all I was interested in was watching *Seinfeld* and *Home Improvement* on the television. That was it. My body had been opened again, this time at my stomach, and I wanted for a moment to forget all about it. I never did get to watch all of the show because the doctors had discovered the source of the problem.

I knew right from the start that the cancer had returned. Before surgery, I had told Dr. Pyne repeatedly that it was cancer, but, being a doctor, he needed to know scientifically. Finally, after testing for pretty much everything he could think of, he found the answer.

My father held my hand as Dr. Pyne came into my little pink private room. He was a big, gentle man, and that day I remember he was wearing red clogs. I gave him one look, and knew exactly what he was going to say.

"It's back, isn't it?" I asked quietly.

"Yes," he told me. "Your cancer has spread."

When I heard those words, I felt like I'd fallen into a different world. I couldn't stop myself. That world of TV nights, of barbecues, of all the simple, normal things I had in my life . . . all gone. That life, that normalcy is so precious. I never realized how much until it was taken away from me.

The cancer I have, a grade four, fast-growing cancer, creates a fluid that builds up over time, filling the lungs and surrounding the heart. It's a cancer that cannot be stopped. Dr. Pyne informed me I would have to start chemotherapy right away. My mother was hurting, trying to come to terms with what was happening. My father and I both burst into tears.

Dr. Pyne left us, and my father held my hand tighter and turned to me.

"I would do anything in the world to change this," he told me. His face was filled with worry and exhaustion. He was so lost. And yet, his voice and eyes were filled with unconditional love. "I would change places with you. I would give my life for yours to go on. What's happening to you is so unfair, my baby girl." I was upset with him for saying that. I needed him in my life as much as he needed me in his. I didn't want him to even suggest trading places with me.

He stayed with me that night, as he did every night I was in the hospital. I'd look over to the corner or the doorway, and my father would be there, wearing his checkered shirt and sweater — grey-green with three buttons down the front. His greyish-black hair would be slightly mussed, and he'd hold my hand until I fell asleep.

I stayed in ICU for over a week. A lot of friends came to see me, and my cousin Marc brought my two young nieces, Emillie and Sophie.

Everyone was so supportive. One night, when I was in severe pain, a nurse came to give me an injection, trying hard to console me. All I wanted to do was wash my hair. So, the next day, with the help of another nurse, she did. One nurse put a blue bowl filled with water under my head, holding my head back like a baby's, while the other gently washed my hair. When they were finished, she carefully put it into a ponytail for me and I put some make-up on. It was important for me to keep myself looking good, even if I was dying.

I kept thinking about a young woman in Cornwall I had heard of who had had two children. During her second pregnancy, she was diagnosed with breast cancer. The pregnancy ran its term, but she died before she got to hold her baby. I started to wonder if that would have happened to me, should my baby have lived. To this day, I still think the pregnancy is what triggered my cancer again. There is such a hormonal shift in a woman's body at that time, and there is a hormonal element to breast cancer. I wanted to ask my gynaecologist, but he died in a car accident right after I was diagnosed for a second time. To this day I still don't know for sure.

Then, it came time to leave. Dr. Pyne warned me that he would be coming that evening to remove the tubes from my body — and that it was going to hurt. Two were in my ribs, stuck into my lungs! I was nervous. And, as promised, at 9 p.m. that night, he arrived. Steph stood in the doorway, watching for him.

"He's coming, Sue," he told me.

I rang for the nurse, desperate for a shot of morphine. I knew he wasn't going to freeze the area, and that I was just going to have to endure the pain. Our friend, Marc Vachon, was beside me, holding my hand. The look on Marc's face when he realized Dr. Pyne's intentions was one of horror, but Marc said nothing. He squeezed my hand, making me feel somewhat calm.

Dr. Pyne turned to me.

"Don't breathe . . ." he said.

That's the last thing I remember.

Dr. Vincent Young became my oncologist. I met him at Ottawa General for the first time and he explained the situation to me. The fact was, chemotherapy couldn't save me, it could only maintain me for a while. Maintain, not save. I was only weeks away from my thirtieth birthday, and suddenly the odds on me seeing my thirty-first was slim to none. I was a terminal case.

The hardest part about dying for me was the people I was going to miss. I didn't want to leave my father, my mother, my family, my friends . . . anyone. The fear of dying is the fear of being taken away from the people you love. It's a divorce you don't want. A parting in which you have no say. And you can't be a con-artist, or sweet-talk your dad into taking you to Dairy Queen to get out of it. It's God's choice. You can cry, you can learn to deal with it, you can fight. But the hardest thing to do is to remain optimistic and keep going.

People would say to me "We could all die tomorrow, getting hit by a car," or such. It wasn't said to be insensitive, but rather with the hope that I might see the positive side to my situation. The problem is, having terminal cancer is like being tied up to a chair, sitting in the middle of the road, watching as a large truck barrels toward you. You can't move. You can't get it out of your mind. Like that truck, the cancer is always there, coming straight at you. All you can do is wait.

The idea of chemotherapy terrified me. And even though I knew it helped some people, as far as I was concerned, chemotherapy equalled death. Chemotherapy means losing your hair, vomiting, drastically losing weight — how do you think positively about that? "Okay, I'll lose some weight, that's a good thing," I told myself. Losing my hair, though? That was the worst. I liked looking good and taking care of my appearance. I was terrified about losing my sex appeal. But what choice did I have?

I arrived with Steph in Ottawa for my first treatment, and once again, I was informed of all the possible side effects. The first drug they were giving me was Adriamycin, also known as The Red Devil. The side effects included fever, chills, low white cell blood count, mouth sores, nausea, and hair loss. I sat with the IV attached to my arm, watching as this red poison began to drip into the main line, moving closer and closer to my vein. I couldn't handle it. I ripped out the IV in a panic. The nurse came over immediately, giving me a sedative. She searched my arm for a vein, preparing to redo the IV, but she was having difficulties finding one. I wasn't surprised — they were probably all hiding. In the end, she managed to attach the IV to my arm once more. And once more I watched as the red liquid dripped into the line. I cried as I felt the poison seeping into my body. Afterwards, Steph took me out, bought me a dress and dinner, hoping to console me.

Fluorouracil, a faint yellow solution, and cyclophosphamide, a clear solution, were the other two medications I had to endure. Side effects included nausea, diarrhoea, heartburn, sores, rashes, appetite loss, dizziness, confusion, weakness, and of course, hair loss. I was to receive four cycles of these three drugs ending in November. All this, and only to *maintain* me.

I had just had my first treatment, and the plan was to head up to Mt. Tremblant for the weekend for my thirtieth birthday. As I packed up the car, I took a look across the street at my neighbour Jack's house, and noticed a police car. That past summer, Jack had been diagnosed with a brain tumour. He had asked me how I had dealt with having cancer. I hadn't yet been diagnosed for a second time, so my attitude was very different.

"I never really thought about it, Jack," I told him. "It was like having a wart removed and I didn't think much of it. I'm fine. I don't really think about it anymore."

As I walked down our drive toward their house that day, Jack's wife Rachel came outside. Jack had just died. It was October 3; my birthday. I had just been re-diagnosed myself, and hearing that blew me away. Another death to cancer, and on my birthday to boot. I wondered whose birthday *I* would die on.

Steph and I went up to Tremblant with Stef and Cathy Kobinger. Everyone was quiet and sad, but kind. We hung out in the village and had a few drinks. That night, I cooked supper. Stef and Cathy gave me a lovely candle holder for my birthday — a sun with three prongs out to the side. I've always believed the sun brings hope and the candle holder was perfect. It was nice to be with these people on my birthday, but I was scared. I wasn't crying at this point, but I couldn't concentrate on anything. I couldn't read a book or sleep.

That night, brushing my hair, I noticed it start to fall over my shirt. And the next morning, long strands lay strewn on my pillow. By Monday, when I washed my hair, I couldn't even brush it after my shower. It was all coming out in the brush. I broke down, falling to my knees by the shower. Steph wrapped a towel around me, then wrapped his arms around me, holding me close.

"Let's call Kelly, and we'll cut it," he said gently.

He was so wonderful, comforting me as he helped me stand. And we called Kelly, Steph's stepsister, and she came over and shaved my head for me.

I had difficulties getting used to the wig. It was dark brown and straight, falling just above my shoulders with a small fringe over my forehead. Friends would come up to me, knowing how uncomfortable I was with it, and try to reassure me.

"You can get away with wearing a wig because you have such a pretty face," they would tell me. I knew their intentions were good, but I got so sick of that comment. "You shave your head," I would think to myself, "then I'll tell you what a pretty face you have."

People were just trying to be kind, but it was almost impossible to console me. I couldn't sleep at nights because my mind was caught up in the idea of dying. I felt like I was slipping away. I didn't understand why God was doing this to me. I would watch television in the middle of the night, from 2 a.m. to 4 a.m., even though poor Steph had to get up early in the morning! I'd do it every night — like clockwork.

I didn't want to be alone, either. I just couldn't handle it. I was driving Steph mad, constantly begging him to stay with me. Even though I was tired, I would watch cooking shows continually, then cook up a storm for Steph when he came home. Alain Vachon, Marc's brother, had given me Bernie Siegel's book, *Peace, Love and Healing: Body-Mind Communication and the Path to Self-Healing*, a week after I got out of the hospital. The problem was, I couldn't even get through a paragraph because when I finished, I couldn't remember what I had just read. While it was a very motivating book, I was so screwed up both physically and emotionally that I couldn't concentrate on it.

I became closer to our friends Paul and Jody Marleau at that time, because Paul had lost his brother Alain to cancer within months of the diagnosis. He had been a young, healthy guy, and he passed away around the time I was re-diagnosed. When I fell asleep at night, I found myself thinking of Alain, wondering if I would go as quickly as he did.

The other side effects from chemotherapy came soon after. My energy levels dropped significantly. A few days after the treatment, my esophagus started burning. Tomatoes, red wine — anything acidic — I could no longer enjoy because of the pain. Then, after a few days of that, I would develop mouth sores. I was given a liquid —

basically another drug — to swish around in my mouth, then swallow. Next, I went through the rollercoaster of being constipated, then having diarrhoea. Not only that, but my body had been thrown into early menopause. Despite all these side effects, I still hoped the chemo would help. I took my pills to help with the nausea. I took the liquid to help with the sores. All food tasted different, then suddenly I couldn't handle food at all. Chemo is about burning and killing everything inside your body. That was exactly what it was doing.

Chemotherapy was continually giving me infections. I was sick of the hospital, sick of being poked at as people desperately searched my arm for veins. One time, I had *three* nurses looking for a vein in my arm all at once. As a consequence of this, I had a portocath installed for easier venous access. It was implanted under my skin, just above my breast. About the size of a loonie, the port septum has a catheter attached to it which is positioned next to the appropriate blood vessel. All my chemo was done through there, but that didn't stop me from requiring needles for other situations.

One time, when I was feeling ill, Roseanne Carr, a wonderful nurse who would come by and check up on me regularly, argued with me, telling me that I needed to be examined. I fought it strongly at the start, but finally agreed. Steph dropped me off at the front door, and I went in. After I was admitted, I noticed the area they had placed me in for observation was right next to the area for patients with illnesses who were immune to antibiotics! I knew if I was exposed to anyone there and got sick, that would be the end of me.

I started screaming for a doctor, telling them I was leaving, begging to be discharged. No one would let me go. I argued, but no one would listen. So, finally, I got up and started walking down the hall. I made it very clear that no one was going to stop me. I informed them firmly that I had a low blood count, and that I should be in isolation.

"I can't be hanging around here," I said when they tried to stop me.

I informed them that I was going home, and that Roseanne could give me my antibiotics there. Finally, a harried nurse found Dr. Pyne, and he agreed to sign me out. So, Roseanne agreed to come by my house three times a day — morning, afternoon, and the middle of the night — to administer my antibiotics by IV.

Roseanne became a close friend, acting as the support system that I needed desperately. She was there every day to listen to me, even if she didn't need to perform any nursing duties. In ways, I became closer to the nurses I got to know than I was to my own friends. They dealt with illnesses every day, knowing things that people outside the profession wouldn't necessarily know. While my friends were most certainly supportive, the nurses understood things on a different level, which I appreciated.

As the winter approached, Steph and I started growing distant again. I knew when the physical affection began to dwindle that once again we were drifting apart. It was the same feeling I had when Rob was in the hospital; Steph was pulling away. He was still taking trips, and working quite hard while I was struggling with depression. I had a nurse from the Red Cross coming in to help me with the house-work, and while I was extremely grateful for her help, it wasn't the company I needed.

Christmas time came, and I truly believed it would be my last. I had started thinking about my funeral arrangements, and had decided on the song "Immortality" by Celine Dion. The line "*We don't have to say good-bye*" made me think of Steph. And one night, listening to it, I had an idea. I wanted to give him a special gift, something he would have to remember me by after I was gone. I sat down and made a special card covered with photographs of us, all cut out in heart shapes. Then, I wrote a poem inside. The final touch involved two gold chains, and a heart trinket that split in two. "Best Friend" was engraved on the back in tiny lettering. The plan was, I would keep half, and he would wear the other. And when I died, he would have both pieces to wear.

"For now, you have half my heart," I told him. "But when I'm gone, you'll have my whole heart. You'll always have my whole heart."

And yet, that Christmas, we sat at opposite ends of the couch, like strangers.

My treatments in Ottawa continued. I had been through four cycles of the previous chemo mix, and now I was taking Taxotere. The physical side effects were the same as the others, only I reacted quite badly to it. As a consequence, the doctors prescribed Benedryl along with it. I was unconscious for hours after my three-hour treatment at the hospital. The hardest part was facing Dr. Young after he examined the results. His head would be down, which I dreaded. I knew what that meant, and I knew how badly he felt. Good news was not on the horizon.

In January, I got a particularly bad infection. I spent all my time in bed with a fever which was growing worse and worse with each hour. I knew I would need antibiotics — again — but I couldn't bear another hospital trip. At this point, I hated the hospital more than anything. So I lay there, with Mission beside me, trying to convince my parents, Tante Denise, and Roseanne that I could last 24 hours. I had a treatment in Ottawa the next day, and I could see the doctor then. There was no need for me to go to the Cornwall ER. So they all gave me a sponge bath, trying to bring down the fever, which continued to rise.

The next day, I went to Ottawa with my aunt and my father. After a few tests, the doctors informed me that I needed to stay overnight. My father tried to get a hold of Steph, but couldn't locate him anywhere. Things between Steph and I were so bad at this point that I hardly ever saw him. I couldn't stop crying as my aunt wheeled me up to admitting. I didn't want to stay overnight, but I was so sick at this point, and terribly nervous. They had seen a spot on my kidney, and wanted to perform another CT scan the next day. Then, they would hopefully know what was going on.

The doctor came into my room the next day and immediately asked me if I had been sexually active with more than one partner.

"No!" I exclaimed, "Look at me! I've got no hair, I'm totally sick!" The fact was, I felt like a monster. My self-esteem was rock bottom at that point.

"You have a urinary tract infection," the doctor informed me. "It has travelled to your gall bladder." A normal, healthy body could have fought it better, but my immune system was too low. Then he told me he asked that question only because one of the causes is multiple sexual partners.

My heart stopped right then and there.

Within a few hours, Steph arrived at the hospital. He leaned against the wall, by the window, keeping his distance. Fifteen minutes later, he left. I lay there, alone and emotionally drained, until nine o'clock that night. Just as I was aching for company, Olga, my cousin Marc's wife, arrived with two cups of coffee and a bag of donuts. Just her being there made me feel so much better. She is a wonderful listener, but she also knows how to talk about nothing for hours. And that was exactly what I needed. We formed the beginning of a bond that night, one that has grown stronger over time.

When I returned home, the arguments continued between Steph and me, sometimes late into the night. Both of us were trying to cope with this insane situation that was pushing us further apart. In the end, I got my doctor to prescribe some sleeping pills, just so I could numb the pain. It was the easiest coping mechanism I had. I could make myself pass out so I didn't have to listen when Steph came home late and wanted to argue. I didn't have to feel anything when he screamed for me to *do something* with my life, rather than just sit at home. If an argument started, and I wasn't prepared, I would reach for the drawer and pull out the pills, claiming I had a headache. Then, I would pass out quietly while he continued to shout. Some nights, I lay there crying and praying silently for a change. For silence.

The chemo continued, and the infection was cured. The spot on my kidney turned out to be nothing. My marriage was still a shambles, and my tolerance level was getting very low. Something had to change.

At home, I had a sheet with dozens of numbers and days and times for different pills and treatments. Everything was arranged like clockwork so I wouldn't miss a beat. And somehow, one day I managed to screw it up. I sat there, staring at the crazy sheet and endless bags of pills, and I marvelled at what my life had become.

"This is stupid," I said. "I don't want to do this anymore."

Joanne Pilon, my good friend, was living in Vancouver at this point. Knowing my condition, she was planning on coming back to Cornwall in order to visit with me. She called me up that night, and as I listened to her, I had a thought. I had never been to Vancouver before.

"No," I said. "You know what? I'm going to come out and visit you."

I had had enough of chemo, of pain, and of emotional distress, and I couldn't handle it anymore.

It was time for an adventure.

CHAPTER FIVE

The Journeys West

Vancouver seemed like the perfect chance to feel normal, if only for a short time. The date was set; the next weekend I would be in Langley with Joanne and her husband, Don.

When Steph got home, I asked him if he wanted to join me on my excursion. He didn't know if he could get the time off, but he clearly wanted to come with me.

"You're either coming or you're not. But I'm going," I told him.

"Okay," he said. "I'll go."

I told my doctor only after we had purchased the tickets and made all the arrangements. I met up with Dr. Young, and told him straight out that I didn't want to do chemo anymore and that I was leaving for a vacation. He knew that there was no more he could do for me anyway. I hated it when he would remind me that chemo was only going to *maintain* me. I wanted him to say that they would do their best to save me, that there were new drugs available . . . that somehow, I would live.

"Go," he said. "When you get back, we'll talk more about the chemo."

Joanne's husband Don picked us up at the airport. After making the 45-minute trip back to Langley from Vancouver, we arrived at the house. Don, Steph, and I relaxed outside with a beer, waiting for Joanne to come home from work. Seeing the mountains, watching the flowers starting to bloom in their garden, it was beautiful. Finally,

Joanne returned, and the boys went off to buy some more beer, leaving us alone. Seeing Joanne was such a relief. There we were, hugging each other, crying, and excited to be reunited. We relaxed in the living room, chatting and catching up, when I asked Joanne if I could show her my head. I wanted to see her reaction — see if she found it repulsive or not.

"Okay," she said.

So I took off the wig, exposing my bald head to my good friend.

"Hey!" she said, smiling, "It's Sinéad O'Connor!"

We laughed at that, and I felt much, much better.

The plan was to spend a few days in Langley and Vancouver, then head up to Whistler/Blackcomb to get some skiing in. Don's boss had a condo there and made arrangements for us to stay in it over the weekend. Joanne and Don could only stay for the weekend, so Steph booked the two of us into the IntraWest condos to get in a couple of extra days of skiing.

For the first few days of our trip, we biked and rollerbladed through Stanley Park in Vancouver with Joanne's two dogs, made wonderful salmon suppers over the barbecue, and enjoyed the exquisite atmosphere. Steph and I were bickering quite a bit, however. I was hoping things would calm down when we got to Whistler.

The skiing was fantastic. After Joanne and Don left, Steph and I settled into a routine. We would ski all day, then have our "happy hour" time — which consisted of a few glasses of red wine — then we would slip into the communal outdoor hot tub where everyone hung out after a day of skiing for a long soak. I kept my blue Nike hat on over my wig the entire time. I had nightmares of my hair flying off my head as I sped down the slopes, so I wore the hat as a precaution. That wasn't the only reason, though. As far as I was concerned, the hat made the wig seem much more natural.

That first evening, sitting there, I realized that two men close by who were also in the tub were staring at me. I shifted, trying to ignore their gaze while people chatted around me.

"Why do you wear that hat?" one of them asked me.

I turned to face the two men. The one who spoke smiled at me, waiting for my response. He asked again, and I kept thinking, My God, who is this guy? I was growing very uncomfortable at his line of questioning. Could he tell it was a wig?

"How come you wear it everywhere?"

I didn't want to answer. Instead, I smiled slightly, and moved to the other side of the tub in order to avoid him.

Of course, my actions only intrigued him more.

The next evening, and two or three glasses of wine later, Steph and I headed down to the hot tub once more. We sat with a small group of people, and Steph started explaining to the others how his inability to smell came from the fact that he had smashed his nose on the bottom of a pool. Suddenly, I noticed the two men from the previous evening nearby. Once again, they were smiling at me.

And once more, the tall man posed the question:

"Are you going to tell me why you always wear a hat?"

I stared at him, annoyed.

"You have pretty hair," he said. "Why would you —"

"It's a wig," I told them. At this point, with the wine flowing through my system, I was feeling a bit more confrontational than usual. "I've lost all my hair from chemo. I don't want my wig flying off when I'm skiing, so I keep it on. I don't want to talk about it because I've accepted things the way they are and that is that!"

He started asking very specific questions about my symptoms, sincerely interested. So, I gave him more details. The first cancer. The second cancer. The fact that I was running away from being poisoned by chemo, and I was sick of doctors telling me they could only "maintain" me, and I was going to die . . . what the hell do they know

anyway? I had decided enough was enough, and it was time to detox-
ify my body, that I was going to take a new route, with acupuncture
and vitamins and . . . and that was it.

"I'm a doctor," he said, completely catching me off guard. He was a
surgeon, specializing in head and neck cancer, searching for a cancer
vaccine at the University of Washington, Seattle. Not only that, but
his friend was also a doctor.

My God, here I was sitting with two doctors and I just finished
bashing the entire medical system. I could have just drowned.

He introduced himself as Doug Villaret, and told me he might
know of someone who could help me. A colleague of his, Dr. Bob Livingstone, was the Chief of Medicine at the Breast Cancer Research
Facility at the University of Washington. Dr. Livingstone was involved
with research for a new drug which targeted certain types of breast
cancer. It was still in the experimental stages, but it was nothing like
chemo, Doug explained. He told me that the doctors in Ottawa had
given up too easily, and he invited me to come to Seattle so he could
get me into a research program for a new cancer treatment.

I wasn't really listening to him at this point. Even though he
claimed it wasn't at all like chemo, I was so fed up with the medical
system, I wasn't interested in listening to anything related to it. Steph,
however, had listened carefully to Doug's story. He invited Doug and
his friend to join us for dinner that evening, which they accepted.

Over dinner, Doug explained that based on my symptoms, I might
just be an eligible candidate for this new drug. The problem was, I
couldn't afford a journey to Seattle. Instead of making a decision
right then, the conversation shifted to include both Steph and Doug's
friend. That night, Doug and I bonded not only as doctor/patient,
but as friends. He was warm and caring, with a generous heart. Any
reservations I had previously suddenly vanished.

Doug was staying in a shared room with the other doctor. Doug's girlfriend, Sarah, was coming up the next day, so Steph invited both doctors and Sarah to stay for a couple of extra days. He arranged for us to move to a larger condo so that all of us would fit in comfortably.

"We can get to know each other better, and you both can get in some more skiing," he said.

Doug agreed, and the group of us moved into a larger condo the next day. Steph and I had a spacious room, as did Doug and Sarah, and the other doctor had a smaller room all to himself. There was a large kitchen in the middle of which we took full advantage. That first night, I made a huge pasta dinner for everyone. It was a lovely evening filled with laughter and conversation.

The topic of Seattle came up again, and I still didn't have an answer. The problem was, I wasn't working, and financially, I didn't think I could pull it off.

"Let me think about it," I told Doug, finally.

Doug appeared in my life on February 3, 1998. I had always believed that three was my unlucky number, but I soon learned differently. As a consequence of this chance meeting, my life was about to change drastically.

Steph and I returned to Cornwall, and fell back into our routine. February 1998 brought with it a brutal ice storm that hit Montreal and surrounding areas in a very serious way. It began as a snow storm, then the weather warmed up, and it turned into rain and slush. A drop in temperature caused the rain to freeze. For three days, freezing rain pelted the area, turning the trees into huge ice sculptures. The trees grew heavy, knocking down power lines and killing the electricity for large communities. People had to be evacuated from their homes and live in community centres until the power had been restored.

Cornwall was hit badly as well, but not to the same degree. Because I was still in my own world, I didn't realize just how serious the storm was. As far as I was concerned, I was still alive, and I wanted to take advantage of that. In ways, I found it fun that we had to have candles everywhere instead of lamps.

As a consequence of the storm, my parents' roof had iced over, and Dad pulled out the ladder, trying to remove some of it. It was then, as he was working, that he suddenly grew short of breath. It was the same thing that had happened to me months earlier.

He went to the doctor, but didn't tell me about it. The next thing I knew, he was scheduled for surgery with Dr. Pyne in the Hôtel Dieu Hospital in Cornwall on February 18. Once I found out, I insisted on going with him.

We arrived at the hospital, only to find out when Dr. Pyne came in that there was a problem. Dad had gotten some of the instructions mixed up. He was supposed to perform an enema the night before by drinking a prescribed liquid, and he forgot to do so. My father started biting the inside of his lip, something he always did when he was nervous.

"Mr. Giroux," the doctor told my father, "we can't do this. You didn't do what you were supposed to do. We're going to have to reschedule the surgery."

I grabbed Dr. Pyne by the arm.

"Please, Dr. Pyne, *please* do it. Don't put my dad through this."

My father was so nervous about the surgery, but he was putting up a brave front. I knew rescheduling it would be hard on him, and I couldn't bear to watch.

Dr. Pyne sighed, gave me a long look, and finally said:

"Okay, I'll do this just for *you*."

Within minutes, a bunch of nurses came in to perform a string of enemas for my father, cleaning him out and preparing him for surgery.

"Dad, you have to do this," I told him.

So, they started the procedure. In the breaks between the procedure, I spoke with him. I started telling him about Whistler, and Doug, and this new treatment . . . and about going to Seattle. Everything Doug had told me.

"Go!" was the first thing he said. "What have you got to lose? You don't meet a doctor in a hot tub that knows somebody who may have a treatment for you every day. It's fate! Go!"

"Really?" I asked. "But I can't afford it."

"Don't worry," he said. "We'll worry about it later."

That was the end of our conversation. The nurses returned, and rolled my father out for surgery. As he headed through the two doors leading into the OR, I told him:

"Bye . . . I love you. It will be fine."

There was a little payphone next to the doors, and I headed straight for it. Without a second thought, I called up Doug in Seattle.

"I'm going to do it," I said.

"That's wonderful! Let me see if I can make an appointment with Dr. Livingstone and I'll call you right back."

"You can't," I explained. "I'm at the hospital. I'll call *you* back."

Within minutes, I was on the phone with Doug again.

"I've got an appointment for you on March 2," he told me.

"Okay," I told him. "I'm going to call the travel agent right now and book it."

I called my travel agent, and booked the entire trip from that small phone booth. Doug would pick me up from the airport and I would stay with him. For the few hours my father was in surgery, I was making plans to go to Seattle. Finally, my mother got off work and joined me at the hospital. Just as I hung up the phone after informing Doug that everything was booked, I saw Dr. Pyne coming out of the OR.

Once again, he was wearing those red clogs, just as he had when he informed me my cancer had returned. It's funny, the things you notice. I can picture him so clearly . . . walking down the hallway, those red clogs clicking on the floor.

"I've got to talk to you," he said.

"*Oh, God . . .*" I whispered.

Mom and I followed him into a little room . . . those infamous *little* rooms. And there, he told us what I had dreaded the most. My father had lung cancer. A fast-growing cancer. He had six months to live. Tops. My father was only 59 years old.

I watched as my mother completely crumpled before my eyes. She just couldn't believe it. First me, and now my dad. I sat there, stunned. It was then that I remembered what he had said to me as I lay in the hospital months ago:

"I would do anything in the world to change this. I would change places with you. I would give my life for yours to go on . . ."

That's what he was doing.

He was just starting to come out from the anaesthesia when Dr. Pyne told him the news. He told Dad straight out: he had six months to live. I don't think my father even cried. He just closed his eyes, as though he knew. As though he was expecting this. As though his prayers had been answered.

I wanted to cancel my trip. The only problem was, when you have cancer, it is impossible to get travel insurance. If I cancelled, I wouldn't get any money back, but I didn't care. All I wanted was to be with my father.

"I booked it," I told him. "But I don't want to go to Seattle anymore."

"Yes, you're going to go," he said firmly. "You'll only be gone for one week. I've got six months, maybe more. This is for you. This is fate. *You have to go.*"

So, the decision was made once more. I didn't cancel. I was going to Seattle in search of a cure.

My mother and I visited him every day. A friend of his, Adele Bray, was also in hospital, staying in the room down the hall. They had been on a few religious retreats together. She owned the Boulerice Funeral Home.

"I want to go see her," I told my parents.

"Why?" my mother asked.

"Dad and I have got to make plans," I said. "We're going to have a double funeral, because he's not going without me. And I'm not going without him. So, let's see if we can be buried in bunk beds, and get a discount!

"You're getting the bottom bunk, because you're heavier," I joked with him. The humour was dark, and designed to cheer my dad up in a sense, but there was an element of truth to my words. The fact was, we were both dying, and funeral arrangements would be necessary. I went to see Adele, and I told her that both my father and I wanted to make funeral arrangements with her once he was discharged from the hospital. My father, however, didn't want to make any plans. He wasn't ready to go there — not yet.

Tante Denise and Oncle Fern were in Florida when they found out about my father. They headed straight back, driving day and night to be by his side. My father had always been close to his large family, and all of them were there to support him. Dad had been discharged from the Hôtel Dieu hospital for a short while, and the time came for his appointment at Ottawa General — the chemotherapy discussion.

Denise and Fern joined my parents and I on the trip to the hospital. Oncle Fern couldn't handle going into the room with us, so he waited out in the hall. The rest of us made our way into another little room. Dad's doctor came in and gave us all the treatment options available to my father. He could be given a mega-high dose of chemotherapy, or it was possible for them to perform surgery once more, which meant taking out a section of his lung. In both cases it would be extremely painful, and there were no guarantees. It would also put my father in bed for a year, which he didn't want. When the doctor was finished, he left us to contemplate the next move.

My father sat there among us, with his decision already made: he didn't want to do anything. And yet, when he opened his mouth to speak, all he could do was cry. He was worried we were going to be angry at him for giving up. He always worried about everyone else first. *I* knew what he would suffer undergoing that treatment. How could I push someone to do it when I had rejected the same treatment myself? My father prayed for strength, and for forgiveness, but as far as I was concerned, he hadn't done anything wrong.

"No, Dad," I told him. "We aren't angry. We love you."

We all started hugging him, letting the tears flow. Finally, the doctor returned, and my father said no to the surgery and to chemotherapy. We respected his decision.

When we got back into the van, I lay down in the back while my aunt drove. The others started talking, but I stayed silent. I let myself grieve as we returned to Cornwall, unable to believe everything that was happening.

February slowly crept closer to March, and I prepared myself for the trip to Seattle. It was a journey to a new city, and the possibility of a new chance for life.

I had no idea what to expect.

Steph drove me to the airport in Ottawa, saw me off, and was going to pick me up a week later. It would be my first time flying alone, and I was nervous about it, even though I saw it as a big adventure. Not only that, but it was such a *relief* to leave Cornwall. Leaving town felt like I had had a million pounds lifted off my shoulders, especially since it was so stressful at home. I just needed a break from the problems with Steph, from the reality of my father's situation — everything. I could have been going anywhere, and I would have been happy. The bonus was, I was going off to do something productive; I was being responsible to myself.

I was carrying all my X-rays with me, along with my CT scan results — I even had to bring my tumour! The first plane I got into was a tiny, tinny thing that looked like a giant bird, and we had to duck to get inside. I was grateful to get into Toronto and change to a more comfortable plane. The minute I finally settled into that plane, I felt relieved and I relaxed.

I started chatting with the woman next to me, telling her my whole story, and my hopes for this adventure. She was on her way to meet with Bill Gates, which I found rather amazing.

"What's he like?" I asked her.

"Oh, just what you'd think," she said. "A real computer guy."

It was a long flight, but a comforting one. When we got to the airport, she helped orient me through customs. Once in the main area, I spotted Doug.

Doug gave me a big hug, taking my suitcase from me. From the airport, he took me down to the Seattle public market for lunch. We wandered around, catching up and enjoying the day. At one point, we stopped at a flower shop, and he went in and bought me a beautiful bouquet of flowers as a welcome present. That night, he invited his girlfriend Sarah and a few of his friends over for dinner.

The next day Doug had to work, so I wandered around Seattle. I did a boat tour, walked along the shore, and took photographs (which never did turn out). It was nice to have the chance to explore on my own. My appointment was the following day, and Doug would be with me, which was comforting. It is always important to have someone in the room with you when you meet a doctor to discuss results and so forth. When you find out you have cancer, your hearing shuts off, and only a few words get through. Depending on your state of mind, it's usually the negative ones — cancer, malignant, death — that you remember afterwards. The rest is a blur. Once you leave the meeting, you realize that you have no idea what the doctor just said. When you have someone with you, they hear what you don't hear, like a personal tape recorder. That way, the meeting hasn't been a total loss. For my meeting with Dr. Livingstone, Doug was my tape recorder.

Doug had seen my CT scans, and his concern came through. The tumour had grown a lot around my heart and lungs. Based on that growth, it appeared as though I only had about a year to live. The problem was, experimental drugs cannot be prescribed until the standard testing procedures had been completed. So, I waited to hear what Dr. Livingstone had to say.

Dr. Livingstone is one of the top oncologists for women in the U.S. He was distinguished for providing expert treatments for women, and is one of the leading clinical doctors for breast, lung, and colon cancer in women. Sitting in his office with Doug, I listened carefully as he explained Herceptin to me. Herceptin was an experimental drug with high prospects. The rumour circulating among the experts in the field was that this could be a "magic bullet"; only, however, if I proved genetically compatible. That meant I had to have a defective Her-2/neu gene.

Dennis Slamon, an American oncologist, and Axel Ullrich, a molecular biologist from Germany, were responsible for pinpointing this gene in 1986. Their research showed that 35 per cent of the breast tumours studied had mutations in the Her-2/neu gene. The mutations cause the breast cells to create abnormal protein levels which work as receptors on the surface of these cells. Working as TV antennas, these receptors receive the chemical signals sent out by the body. Once received, the cells are stimulated to grow — but with so many proteins, they start to grow out of control. So, after isolating this gene, Dr. Slamon and Dr. Ullrich managed to isolate a monoclonal antibody that was attached to the protein, and by doing so, managed to create Herceptin. Herceptin wasn't designed to kill the tumour, but to prevent further growth with possible shrinkage.

The question became, was I eligible for this new drug?

Herceptin was being manufactured in the U.S. by Genentech at the time, but was expensive and complicated to create. Also, there were no guarantees that it would work. Because breast cancer activists had found out about this new drug, a lot of pressure had been put on Genentech to create a compassionate release program for terminal patients, even though the drug was still in the second phase of testing. Releasing Herceptin to all the women with the Her-2/neu deficiency was impossible, and yet there was a large amount of pressure on the company. Finally, in 1995, they agreed to a compassionate release program to small groups of individuals. To avoid being accused of favouritism, they created a lottery system where 25 eligible women would have their names drawn every four months and they would receive Herceptin treatments at no cost. Twenty-five women. Of thousands.

Dr. Livingstone explained that the next step would be to test my tumour for this gene. My doctors in Ottawa would have the results in a couple of weeks. I knew that a breast examination was coming up. I was starting to get tense, because Doug was still in the room. Soon, I could hardly hear what Dr. Livingstone was saying to me. I knew Doug was a doctor, so feeling nervous was silly, and yet, he was now a friend too. But just before the examination, he left without my having to say a word.

Later, when I spoke with Doug, he told me it wasn't Herceptin he had been thinking of when he recommended I come to Seattle for tests. And yet, at this point, I didn't care what it was, so long as it wasn't chemotherapy.

I had a wonderful time while I was in Seattle. Doug had planned things for us to do every night I was there. One night, we saw a show. Another night, we went to a charity casino event following the classic "thirties" style. Everyone was dressed in costume. Men ran around dressed as Keystone Cops swinging their billy clubs. We had shopped that afternoon, searching for a big hat for Doug, as well as some other clothing for our costumes that evening. The money gambled was play money. At the end, the idea was to pool your winnings together to purchase tickets towards winning a cruise vacation. Unfortunately, we didn't know that, and instead gave our money away! Another time, we drove around Seattle, seeing where the movie *Sleepless in Seattle* had been filmed. Then we went shopping, and Doug bought me the movie. I spent one afternoon just looking at pictures with Doug, learning all about his life.

I made a few calls to the house, but I never got in touch with Steph. I was concerned about Mission, wanting to make sure that he was being fed and walked. I spoke with my parents every night. I wanted to ask my father to check up on the dog, but I didn't want to add anymore stress to his life, considering what he was going through.

My last day, I spent with Joanne, who had driven down the coast from Vancouver just to see me. We spent an amazing day together, wandering around Seattle. During our time together I told her I had this weird feeling that Steph wouldn't be at the airport to pick me up when I arrived home.

"As if," she said.

When I spoke with my father before leaving, he felt it too.

"Why don't you have Marc and Olga pick you up at the airport?" he said, his tone serious.

"No, Dad," I said, "He said he's going to be there, and he'll be there. Don't worry about it."

I didn't want to phone Steph up and tell him it was okay if he wasn't there. We were having so many problems as it was, I didn't want him thinking I didn't trust him. I just wanted to leave it alone, and give him the benefit of the doubt.

"You're going to be tired, you're coming in late, you're going to be on Seattle time, it's a long flight, and you're not well and your system is still down and —"

"— Dad, it's okay. It's okay."

I hung up the phone, and Doug agreed with my father.

"Why don't you call your cousin Marc and have him pick you up from the airport?" he said.

"No, no," I said. "It'll be fine."

The next day, Doug's friend drove me to the airport, because Doug had a 12-hour surgery scheduled for that day. And all the way there, I had that same feeling . . . Steph wouldn't be there to pick me up. In my head, I kept trying to imagine that he would show up with roses and open arms. Sitting on the plane, listening to my walkman, I stared out at the sky, my faint reflection showing the big tears rolling down my face.

Sure enough, when I got to the airport, I came out of the first door and looked around for him — and there was no one there. I phoned home, but there was no answer. I called his best friend, but he didn't know where Steph was. So, I called his secretary for Steph's cell phone number because all of a sudden, I couldn't remember anything. There was no answer on his cell. Steph was nowhere to be found. I was so upset at this point, I called my father-in-law, Pierre, the only person left I could think of. My calm had completely vanished as I hysterically told him the situation. Afterwards, I apologized.

"I'm just very frustrated," I told him.

"Just stay there. I'll come pick you up."

"Forget about it," I said. "It'll take you another hour to get me and I've already been here an hour. I'm just going to grab a cab home."

I went to the bank machine and pulled out about $200. The cab dropped me off at Pierre's house, because I didn't have a house key on me. The ride set me back $125, and I got out, exhausted and drained.

Pierre drove me to the house and opened the door for me. Once inside, I started to rant again. Pierre just sat on the couch and looked at me. He didn't say a word, he just let me vent, which I appreciated. Once I finished, we were finally able to reach Steph through his cell phone. His father told him to get his ass over to the house. Steph phoned back right away, telling his father that it was all right and that he should go back home.

"Don't leave, Pierre," I begged. "He'll start yelling at me and again it will be my fault. Please don't. I want to sleep in peace."

Steph called a couple of times before getting home, but Pierre stayed. Once he got there, Steph passed out on the couch downstairs. Pierre left soon after, and I made my way up to our bed.

Not even home a full day, and things had gone back to normal.

CHAPTER SIX

One Day at a Time

The next morning, I came downstairs as if I had already accepted what had happened and moved on. Steph was extremely kind, doing everything he could to make up for the previous evening. Once more I was creating this imaginary husband — the Steph of my dreams. The one that I wanted. The husband who loved me, who was happy with me, who would stand by me. The best friend with whom I had things in common. Steph wasn't that person, but I didn't want to start all over again. No one in my family had ever been divorced, and I didn't want to be seen as a failure or let anyone down. I wanted to believe we could work at it and fix our relationship.

The following Saturday, Steph went out to help a friend do some work. He bought me a coffee in the morning and left. Based on a couple of conversations we had during the day, I was starting to doubt that he was where he told me he'd be. I spoke to him about five minutes before he got home, and he asked me to draw him up a bath and make him a martini. When he came in, he was polite but distant. He changed out of his clothing in the laundry room, left his stuff there, then hopped in the bath. At this time, I was "Detective Sue" on a regular basis. I was almost going crazy trying to find out what Steph was up to. I wanted him to admit to me that he was cheating with someone else. So I went into the laundry room and looked through his clothing.

I found a gas receipt that supported my suspicions. I marched into the bathroom, clicked the lights on, and confronted Steph.

"I *cannot* handle this anymore! It's ONE thing after another! I asked you a week ago if you wanted to work this marriage out and you told me you wanted to and I told you we can't do that if you don't break up with your girlfriend! You *can't have three people in a relationship!* How can you work it out with me if you run to another person every time I do something that *you* dislike?! You CAN'T!"

I couldn't believe those words were coming out of my mouth. I marched right out of the room before Steph could say anything, grabbed Mission, put him on his leash, and stuck him in the back of our pickup truck. I got inside, locked the doors, and started backing out of the driveway. Steph came outside, running after me with only a towel on. I was laughing and crying all at once as he chased me down the road.

In the side pockets of the car door, I found a bunch of cell phone bills with the phone numbers recorded along with the dates and times of calls. I noticed one recurring number in particular, and so I called it.

A woman answered. A young woman.

I told her that I had a message from Steph. I told her she could have him, and I was no longer interested in being with him. Then, the anger bubbled up inside of me.

"What kind of person would have an affair with a man knowing his wife was *dying*?! You have *no compassion!*"

She started telling me that Steph was going through a hard time as well, and needed someone. She told me that I had no idea what he was going through.

I hung up.

I didn't want to hear it, but I knew there was truth in her statement. It grew late, and I found myself driving home. The fact was, I didn't want to be seen as someone who gave up quickly. I didn't know what to expect when I came inside, but all Steph did was hug me. That night, lying in bed, he held me so close, and I couldn't stop crying. Finally, I had to take two sleeping pills in order to fall asleep.

The next morning, April 18, I let myself slip into routine, still hurt, but burying it for the meantime. We were getting ready to go golfing, and there I was, acting as though nothing was wrong. Steph was sitting at the kitchen counter, and I stood opposite him in the kitchen.

And all of a sudden, the façade fell away.

"I can't even look at you," I said. "We're acting as though everything's okay again!"

Finally, I made the decision.

"I can't do this anymore. I'm done. It's over."

I snatched up Mission again, because at that moment, he seemed like the only thing in the world that was mine, and I stormed out. I realized, you can't make someone love you. It has to be mutual. Forcing a relationship will not bring happiness.

After putting the dog in the car, I drove to the corner store. I called up Jody Marleau, my social worker friend who was familiar with the situation. She and I went back to my house to pick up some of my clothing, then went to her place to join Paul and the kids.

I spent the afternoon there, watching Paul read to his two children before they went out to play with the dog in the back yard. I found it so ironic that on this day I would be here, of all places. Jody had everything I wanted: a nice guy, a little boy and girl, the picket fence, the nice house, the in-ground pool . . . it was picture perfect, like a movie. Normal. And I looked at my own life, and saw a woman whose marriage was falling apart, whose father was dying of cancer, and who had cancer herself.

Could it get any worse? I felt totally discouraged.

That night I had dinner with Jody's family, then got up the courage to call my parents and tell them what had happened with Steph. I explained the situation, yet I couldn't commit to saying I was leaving him for good.

"I'm just taking time away from Steph. I need to take a break."

"Okay," my father said. "Come on over."

The worst part about leaving the house was being in a different place and sleeping alone. I wanted someone to hug me so badly that night so I asked my mom to sleep with me. She lay down beside me, and my father joined us. All three of us snuggled close on my bed. I couldn't bear the thought of being alone. I felt like a five-year-old who could only fall asleep if she had her teddy bear.

The next day, I phoned up Steph and told him I was going to stop by the house and pick up a few things with my aunt Denise. I walked in the house, and the first thing I noticed was the absence of the little stereo that Steph and I had just bought.

Once more, I snapped.

"Oh, yeah?" I said quietly. "You're taking the little stereo?"

Right then and there, I called my lawyer.

"What are my rights?" I asked her.

"Take everything you can, because you won't get anything else again. Just take it and get out of there."

So, I called up Rick, cousin Sylvie's husband, and he drove over in his bread truck. Friends of mine showed up to help and we just loaded everything in. I took the kitchen cupboards, my clothes, furniture — everything I wanted. Whatever Steph had purchased before our marriage, I left behind. Then, I drove it over to my parents house for storage.

My neighbours claimed that when Steph got home, they could hear him screaming from the end of the street.

I had a treatment in Ottawa that afternoon. I was continuing with the chemo because at this point I had no other alternative. Dr. Young had also given me a hard time for skipping out on my treatments. It was the middle of April at this point, and my doctor had received the news from Doug regarding my breast cancer.

I had the defective Her-2/neu gene. I was eligible for Herceptin.

The only problem was, I couldn't just march across the border and get treatments. The only chance I had was the lottery for terminal patients. So, when Dr. Young asked me if I wanted to submit my name, I agreed. After all, I had nothing to lose. My final cycle of chemo would be in May, and from there, it was only a matter of time.

Away from Steph, I made a decision to try and make up with Jodi Lyn. She was now working at a funeral home, still singing when she could. I knew she was angry with me for not believing her, but the moment I walked into her apartment, tears filled her eyes. I took off my wig, showing her what I had become, and she hugged me close. We cried, laughed, and bonded all over again that night. I told her how I was close to the end of my rope and how hurt I was about Steph, and she listened like the true friend she was. I ended up staying there all night.

My friendship with Doug grew after I left Steph. We'd call each other regularly. Three weeks after I returned from Seattle, Doug phoned me with sad news. His mother had just been diagnosed with cancer. We were both living with the fear of losing a parent. Our common situations brought us closer together.

It was tough hearing people telling me to stay positive. You want to think that way, and yet you spend your time reassuring those you love who believe that you are going to die soon. With my father being ill, I suddenly saw things from both sides of the fence. I loved my father, and I knew he was going to die, but I didn't want him to give up. He could relate to me like no one else at that point, because we were both suffering from the same illness.

Dad's cancer had been caused by exposure to asbestos in the mill where he had worked 25 years before. Asbestos takes over 20 years to take effect in the body. Tante Denise started questioning the cause of Dad's cancer. She called up the government, asking questions about the rights of workers and asbestos in the hopes that a pension could be obtained for my father from the company. One day, while my aunt was out with my father, a government representative returned her call and gave the details to my uncle. Eventually, a settlement was reached with the people who owned the mill. Meanwhile, the rest of us tried to keep Dad's spirits up.

My father's temper got out of whack as a consequence of the illness. He would snap at little things more often than not.

"Woah, Nellie!" I would say. "Wooooaaaaah!"

Nellie became his nickname. Sometimes, I would sing him a song that I knew would make him giggle. I took the theme song from the *Beverly Hillbillies*, and adjusted the lyrics to suit him:

"Let me tell you a story about a man named Claudie. . . . So the first thing you know, ole' Nellie's a millionaire and the king would say 'MOVE AWAY FROM THERE.' Said Cornwall's not the place you want to be, so they packed on up and moved to Florida."

Laughter and fun were what I wanted for my father. I also wanted him to get motivated, to take care of himself. I didn't want him to give up on me. At this point, I was focused on detoxifying my own body. For that, I went to my friend Mary Bard. I had met Mary and her husband Roger through Steph a year before I was diagnosed the second time, when we went to visit them at their chalet in the Laurentian Mountains. While Mary was also a dental hygienist, we were introduced because Roger had been doing some work for Steph. They were the closest couple I knew, cuddling like they were 16-year-olds on a first date.

Mary became my Dr. Mom. She asked detailed questions about my diet, and made sure I was on the right vitamins — multiple B, C, calcium, magnesium, flax seed oil, anti-oxidants. Not only that, but she got me to read different "healing" books that covered both the

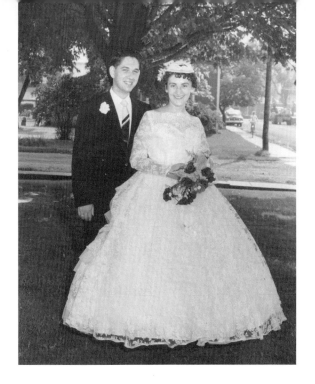

My parents on their wedding day. The day before he
died, my father asked to see this picture so he could
look at his beautiful wife.

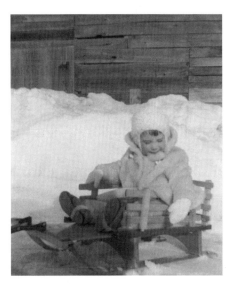

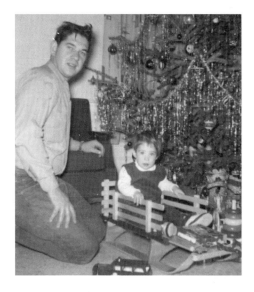

Growing up on the farm, my father would
pull me around in a sled so I could be with
him all day long.

Daddy's little girl.

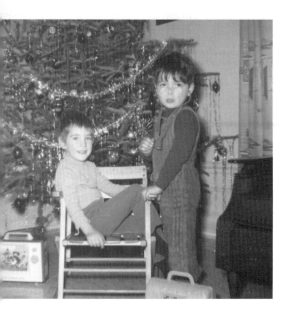

Playing with my cousin Marc.

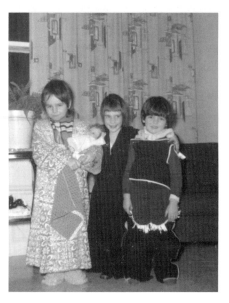

Me with my cousins Sylvie and Marc, playing dress-up.

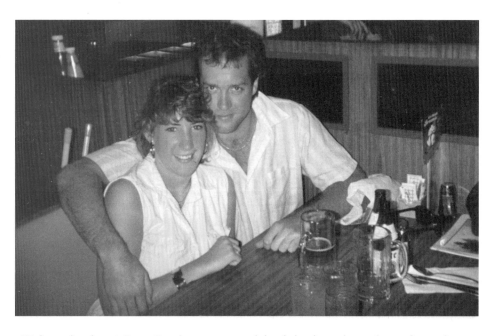

With my first fiancé, Steve. Steve's experience with his father brought me face to face with my own feelings about losing Dad.

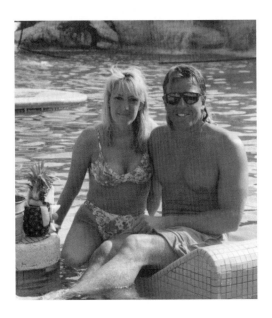

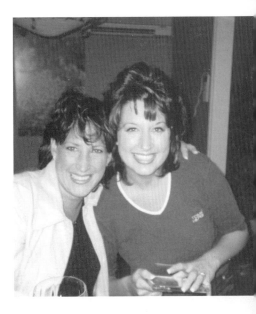

With Rob in Cancun. My dream life ended the day I lost him.

Sharing a laugh with my good friend Jodi Lyn.

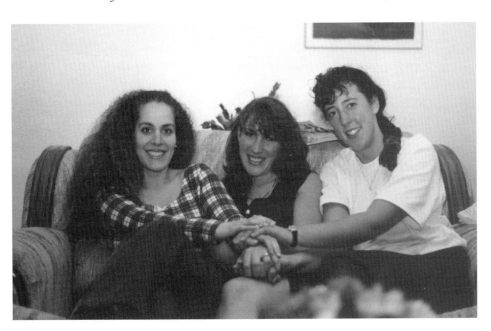

Friends for life: Rita and Joanne.

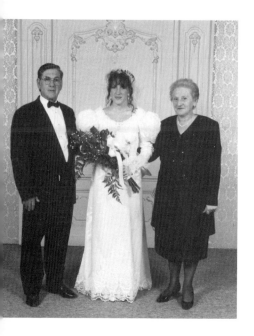

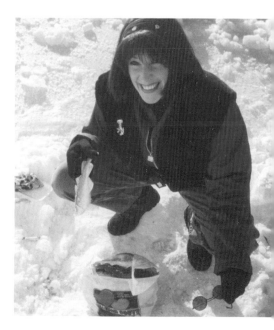

With my parents on my wedding day.

Ice fishing in northern Quebec.

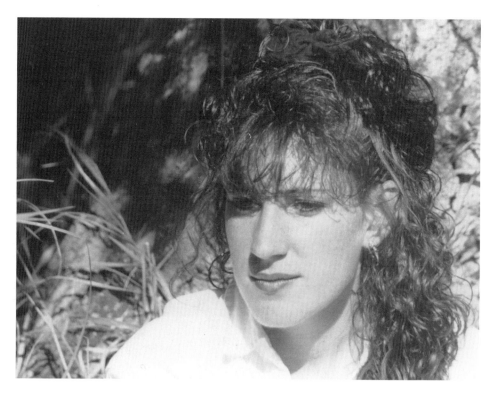

The photo that ran with the *National Post* profile. It would appear that my life was calm and peaceful when this picture was taken; it was anything but.

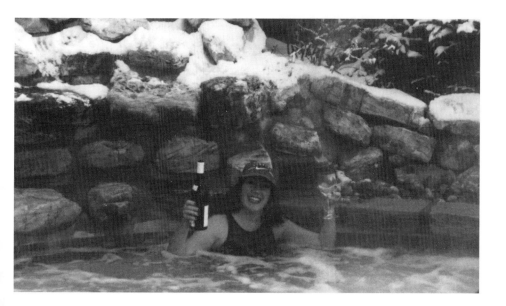

In the hot tub at Blackcomb/Whistler, wearing my wig and Nike cap. I was about to meet someone who would change my life.

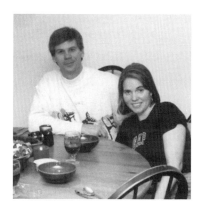

Dr. Doug Villaret and his girlfriend Sarah at our condo in Blackcomb.

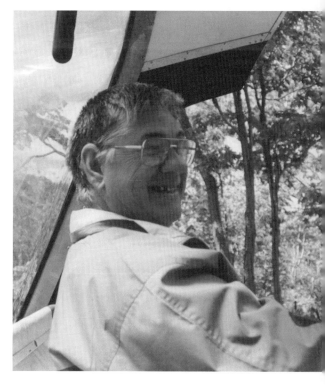

I took this picture of my dad while we were on a chair lift in Mont Tremblant celebrating Father's Day.

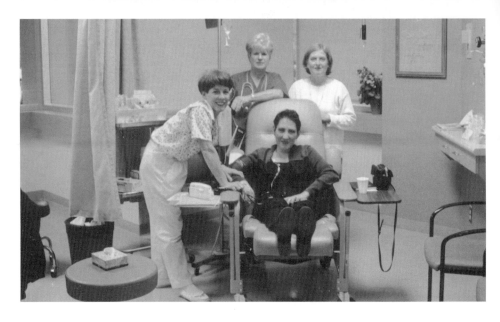

Me and my "nightingales" at the Ottawa cancer clinic.

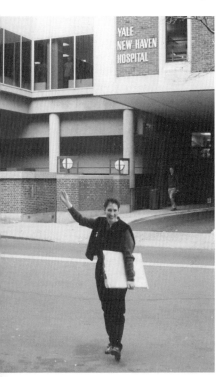

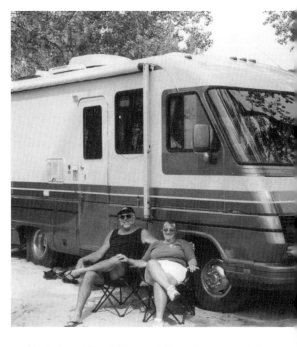

My beloved Oncle Fern and Tante Denise, and the
motorhome that got us to Connecticut and back
for my treatments.

With my medical records in
hand, I'm about to enter the
Yale-New Haven Hospital for
my first Herceptin treatment.

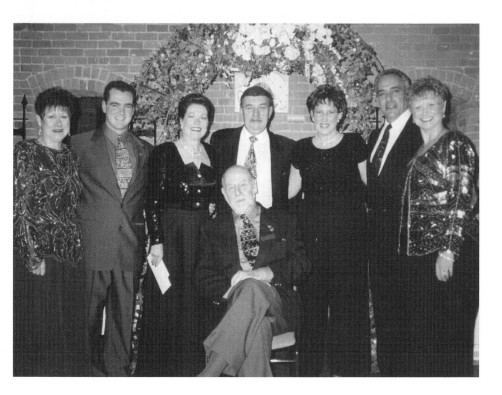

My Chance for Life committee: Barb George, my cousin Marc, Mary Bard, John Ciarlo, me, Rick Kalil, Charlene Charboni, and one of my guardian angels, Ray Matthey, in the front.

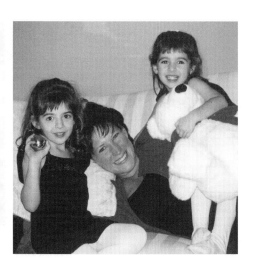

My Disney babies, Emillie and Sophie.

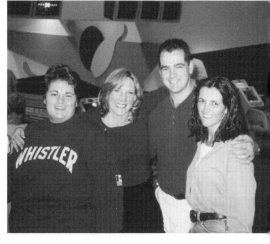

With my cousins, Sylvie, Marc, and Manon: the siblings I never had.

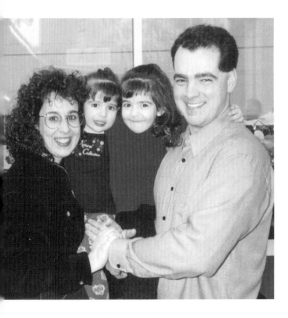

Olga and Marc with my beautiful nieces.

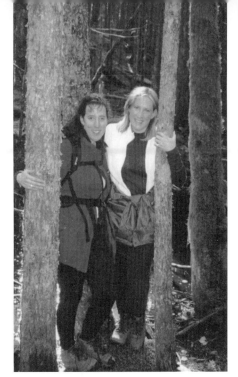

Hiking in BC with Joanne. A new start, with
support from old friends.

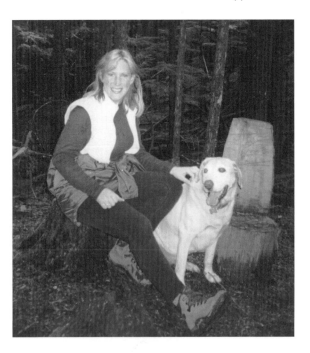

With my Valentine's gift from Rob, Mission.
He's my rock and constant companion.

physical and the spiritual. She also had me exploring alternative therapies — lymphatic drainage, reiki, even acupuncture. While the others I stuck with for quite some time, the acupuncture was only a brief stint. I had had enough of needles. I started working with a massage therapist, Joy Clinton. Like Roseanne, she became a listening ear for me: an undercover angel. Upon her suggestion, I started working with visualization techniques. Keeping focused on healing, that was my goal.

My father, on the other hand, loved his Dairy Queen, his creamy mashed potatoes with lots of butter, and his Kentucky Fried Chicken. While we could mix Ensure and other vitamins with the ice cream and potatoes, the KFC was certainly not good for him.

"Dad, you can't eat that!" I would say.

"What's it gonna do, give me cancer?" he'd joke back.

So he'd pick up the fattest piece of chicken, and dip it in thick gravy, all the while looking at me.

"I'm not eating that stuff," I said, annoyed. "I'm not!"

I really was mad at him. I kept trying to motivate him, stop him from giving up.

"No," he'd say to me, "I'm letting go. Just let me have fun!"

I kept pushing at him to read the same Bernie Siegel book I had been given. I worked hard at changing his attitude, and the book was meant to inspire patients . . . I thought it might do the trick.

"How many pages did you read today?"

"Two," he'd say.

"That's not good enough! You should read a chapter a day, and then you'll get through it!" And he'd try. I could see him taking the book, starting to read, and then falling asleep in his chair.

"HEY!" I would shout. "Read the book! Motivation!"

And yet, I remember when I first was diagnosed, reading was almost impossible. He did try, though, for me.

We started talking to each other, because we were in the same situation. Sometimes it feels like no one can understand what you're going through unless they've gone through it, too. The two of us would be in our separate rooms at night, but both our minds were working overtime. At three in the morning, we would get up because neither of us could sleep. Always three, like clockwork. Dad would join me in my room, and we'd have our talks. We were sharing the same fears — I was scared of losing him, but I was also afraid of dying. It was the same for him. Two different fears for each of us, and all due to one disease.

We would talk about heaven, and he told me how he felt about the idea of losing me. We were living a strange race for time. It was as though we were walking the same path towards the finish line, only I had a head start. My father worked at pulling me back at first, then he joined me. Now, we were walking side by side.

After our talk, we'd turn on the TV and Dad would lie down beside me. We'd watch whatever was on at three in the morning. There was a program called *How Did They Do That?* which would explain how different mechanisms worked, or how certain feats were accomplished. Always, they would say:

"And *how* did they do that?"

There was never a show on the cure for cancer, though. And that was what I wanted the most.

It was June — Father's Day — and Joanne was down from Vancouver visiting with us. It was one of those hot summer days, and since I was living at the house, and not working, I tried to help out as much as I could. Cutting the lawn was one of my jobs. I would wear my walkman, listening to Rod Stewart and singing along.

"If I knew then what I know now . . ."

I would sing it loudly, making sure my father heard me as he watched from the sunroom, rocking back and forth in his little rocking chair.

"You're nuts!" he'd call out.

"It's almost happy hour . . ." I would call back. "Do you want a Caesar?"

"O-kay," he would say.

One Caesar, and he was a happy guy.

Today was different, though. My father started by staring at me from the sunroom as I mowed the lawn, but that wasn't good enough. He came outside and sat on this little barrel, crossing his arms, and studying me carefully. I stopped the mower.

"What are you doing? Would you go inside?" I told him.

"I'm watching you cut the grass to make sure you cut it right."

"Dad," I said, "I've been living here all my life, and I've been cutting the grass for years."

That didn't stop him. He started giving me pointers, telling me how to manoeuvre the mower properly, and so forth. It was a large property, around an acre, and there were a variety of techniques to use when cutting it.

"Dad," I finally said, "Why are you doing this?"

"Well, when I'm gone," he replied, "I want you to do it right. I won't be here to help you out."

Before I could respond, he stood up.

"Come, come," he said. He made me follow him to the garage with the lawn mower in order to show me how to mix the gas, and show me what went with what, and as he did this, I burst into tears. I pulled him close to me, and hugged him tight. As silly as it might have seemed to be crying over a lawn mower, it was the fact that he knew he was leaving. And so did I.

That afternoon, I pulled out a camcorder and Joanne and I joked with my father, wishing him Happy Father's Day! We tried to forget about what he was going through, and worked on cheering him up. My cousin Nicole's little boy, Marco, insisted on coming over to visit with my father. They had a tradition of sharing a small Coca-Cola together. So, sure enough, Marco marched up the hill with Oncle Robert, sat down on Dad's lap, and they shared a Coke on Father's Day.

Later, my mother and I got into the pool, watching as my father walked down the path towards us. My father would always dive straight into the pool, but not today. Instead, he carefully climbed down the ladder, taking baby steps into the water.

"My, God . . . it's so cold . . ." he said.

Right then, he started crying. We all followed suit. I realized for the first time that he was moving ahead of me in our journey to the finish line. He was losing the battle by winning the race.

Dad turned to me, as though just realizing that this was going to be his last Father's Day. Then, he started talking about his father, and how he felt when his dad died at age 49 of cancer.

"It doesn't change," he said. "I still feel the same about it as I did when I was younger."

Dad was quite emotional that day. And while heavy topics were discussed, it was still special. It meant a lot . . . to both of us.

Seeing as I wasn't working, I decided to preoccupy myself by taking a biology correspondence course. Most of my days were spent on the computer in the basement, just doing homework and research. It was the first time I ever got a 98 per cent in anything. It was due, of course, to the amount of time I put into it. That's all I did. My father would come downstairs while I was working.

"Why don't you come upstairs and spend some time with me?" he would ask.

So, I'd grab my work and head upstairs. I'd read my research on evolution out loud . . . and he would fall asleep.

The fact was, he was sleeping all the time, even though he wasn't on treatment. His exhaustion grew as the days went on. The tumour had started to grow on the side, and was causing him discomfort. I would rub ointment on it, massaging it in, hoping to ease the pain, but it wasn't working as well anymore. So, his doctors recommended he do a few chemotherapy treatments in the hopes that it would temporarily solve the problem. After three treatments, the doctors decided it wasn't working, so we just let it go.

My father was a very religious man. Every morning, Tante Denise and Oncle Fern would come over for coffee. They would talk with my dad for a while, and after they left, my father and I would sit on the couch and do the rosary. Every day, three times a day, we would do a rosary. At the beginning, I told him I didn't want to do it, but I saw how important it was to him. It wasn't that I wasn't religious, it's just very repetitive.

"Our father, who art in heaven . . ."

The whole prayer. For each bead on the rosary necklace. And three times a day. One in the morning, one in the afternoon, and one in the evening. Dad would come find me as soon as it was time.

"Sue? Sue, do you want to come and do another rosary?"

I'd either say "No, I think I'll pass on it today," or I would just go. It helped ease my father's mind.

In the evenings, at around seven o'clock, my uncle Robert, who started B & M Meat Market with Dad, and Dad's cousin, Oncle Conrad, would show up. Sometimes their wives, Janet and Helen, would join them. They would chat away, which was great for my father who loved the company. The problem was, it put a lot of strain on my mother. As my father had made the decision to die at home, the house was constantly filled with people wanting to visit him. There was hardly ever a break. It was like living in a hospital. It was a sacrifice my mother was willing to make, giving up her privacy, even though she never had her own space.

Once, Dad and I were both suffering from fevers. Mom raced back and forth, from one room to the next, bringing us pain pills, mopping our brows. She was exhausted mentally, physically, and emotionally. The strain was enormous.

When I think about her during those days, I think about her being lost in a different world. She was working at the Red Cross at this point, but when she was home, she would walk around in circles, constantly repeating that she had to clean the house. Clean clean clean. We were all trying to get as close as possible to my father, but she kept her distance. A lot of times, she would go out into the garage to weep.

I found her out there one day. She was hysterical, crying her eyes out.

"What's wrong? What can I do? Let me help!" I kept saying over and over.

"Go away . . . go away," she repeated.

"Look! I'm living with this too! I have cancer. C'mon, help me here! What can I do?!"

I was going through my own strain, feeling as though I had to take charge at times. When you are dealing with a major illness, it's common to lash out at those who are closest to you, because it's easier than accepting the truth of the situation. You want to blame someone, just to relieve yourself of the pain. I was blaming my mom in my own way, but it wasn't her fault this was happening. She didn't say a word in response. She never took a day off from it, never got a chance to breathe. I wanted to help, but I didn't know what to do. I was so worried about her that I phoned Père Denis Vaillancourt, our family friend and the priest she worked for. He came straight over.

We had a special book, *Reflections and Prayers from the Valley of the Shadow of Cancer* by Eleanor Bouwman, which gave different types of prayers for different times during cancer: when you have pain, when you feel like you're dying, when you've lost hope, etc. There was a whole variety. So, I picked through the book until I found one that worked for how I felt. I lay beside my dad, who was sleeping in his room. He squeezed my hand as I read to him.

My battle to stay positive was waning. Every night, I shut my blinds and was in bed by seven o'clock, watching TV in my room and crying. It was July, and I was extremely depressed at this time, starting to face all the truths I didn't want to face. My marriage had fallen apart, my dad was deteriorating fast, I wasn't working . . . what was there to live for?

Everyone I knew was buying me books. Oncle Conrad's wife, Helen, brought a special journal over. She had also gone through breast cancer and was doing her best to comfort me. Yet, no matter what anyone tells you, it is up to you and you alone to get out of that rut. Each day I was supposed to write down three good things that happened to me that day. What could I possibly think of that made me happy? Nothing. I couldn't think of one thing. It was horrible. So I never wrote in it. I couldn't see the gifts in life.

"One day at a time," the poem inside read. *"That is enough. Do not look back / And grieve over the past because it is gone. . . ."*

One of the biggest problems I was having involved accepting the situation with Steph. I couldn't let go. I knew this wasn't helping me to heal, but it didn't stop me.

It was July 29, the heart of summer, and that evening my parents decided to go to the casino in Ottawa. They begged me to come with them, but I didn't want to. I was feeling completely down at this point. I began drinking. And drinking.

I lost it.

I called up Steph, crying my eyes out and telling him I knew everything that had happened during our marriage. I was hysterical. I knew that he wanted to reach out to me, too. It wasn't easy for him, having a wife who was dying. He must have sensed the condition I was in, because he sent a police officer over to the house to check up on me. I acted as sober as I could, pretending everything was fine. After the officer left, I fell deeper into depression. I was hooked on sleeping pills at this time, so I started popping them like candy. Then, I called the hospital up under the guise of phoning for "a friend."

"I think my friend took too many Tylenols," I said. "How many would she have had to take if it were to kill her?"

I wouldn't give them my name, and they wanted me to come in and talk to them. Finally, I thanked them and got off the phone.

I started writing letters to my cousins, trying to decide what I should leave each of them. So, I wrote a letter to Sylvie, then to Manon, then Marc. I wrote to Tante Denise, and Oncle Fern, and my other cousins, Nicole and Marie. I gave each of them a special piece of jewellery. Then, I wrote a letter to my parents and one to Steph. At that point, I knew what I was going to do. That was it for me. I was done.

I had decided to drive the car into the garage, put some music on, and let it run. I even brought my bottle of wine with me. When I backed up the car, I ripped off the side mirror.

"Oops," I said. Then I remembered I wouldn't even be here to deal with it the next day. I continued backing up. In the process of plowing in like a bulldozer, I smashed the barbecue in the garage, and shattered a glass table. Finally, I closed the garage door, and fell asleep.

The worst part was yet to come.

I found myself waking up an hour or so later. Maybe the garage door wasn't closed. Maybe there was air escaping. Maybe it was the car using recycled gas. Whatever it was, it saved my life. My parents had returned from the casino, and were sitting in the living room when my father suddenly jumped up and headed outside to the garage. When he found me, he started crying, and I followed suit.

"I'm sorry, I'm sorry . . . I didn't mean to do this . . ." I said over and over.

"Why are you doing this? Why? What's going on with you?"

I didn't go to the hospital because I didn't want anyone to know what I had attempted to do. I made my father promise not to say anything. Then, I just went to bed. My parents stayed by my side, both of them sleeping with me that night. Later, my mother asked my father how he knew to look in the garage.

"I had a premonition," he told her.

The next day, they phoned Jody Marleau, as she was a social worker. Jody talked with both my father and I on the phone. Tante Denise came over to spend some time with my father. I had reached my lowest point. There was nowhere to go but up.

That's when things started changing for me. I was seeing life in a totally different way. Things got better and better because now I was accepting my own death. It was my father's death that I couldn't accept. Watching him go and losing my husband at the same time had just pushed me to the edge. So, cleaning up was the first step. I cut out all the sleeping pills, and quit taking Tylenol 3's cold turkey. It was time to take control of my own destiny.

I asked Jodi Lyn to help me with my funeral arrangements, seeing as she was working in one of the homes. I wanted it done right. The theme would be white roses. No carnations, no lilies, just roses all over my casket. The casket interior would be burgundy. Celine Dion would be playing in the background. I went into details with her about what I wanted to wear and what she had to do. It was difficult because she was my best friend, but she agreed. She promised not to burn my skin when she curled my wig, and she promised to make me look like an angel.

It was August 10 — just over a week after my suicide attempt — when I received the call. It was Dr. Young's assistant nurse, Rock.

"Suzanne, you won the lottery!"

I had no idea what he was talking about. The 6/49? It was quite bizarre. I must have been a little dazed at the time.

"How did you get my numbers?" I asked.

"No, no. You put your name into the lottery for Herceptin, and you just won!"

He explained that I would have to go to Texas once a month to partake in the Herceptin study. The Herceptin was supposed to be on a weekly basis. There would be one treatment there, then the other three treatments would be in Ottawa.

I was so excited! All the information was going to be sent to me, and I would receive a phone call with the final details. I went into my father's room, still feeling the rush of excitement from the phone call. He was quite ill at this time, often spending his days in bed. I told him that I had just won the chance to have this new treatment! No more chemo! And then, it hit me. I suddenly realized that I had been given a chance for life. It was the second chance that my father wouldn't even come close to having.

I burst into tears, hugging him close.

My father smiled, as though he knew. He knew that this was the plan God had made for us. It was exactly what my father wanted. Then, we started discussing the details of the treatments. There was a reality to face.

"Dad," I began, "Okay, I won the Herceptin, but we have no money. I'm not working, you're not working . . . how am I going to afford to go to the States? I can't just fly to Texas on a whim, you know?"

"Don't worry," he said. "Everything will come together. Don't worry."

The chances of winning the treatment were so rare, I couldn't bear the thought of not being able to take it. So, I went down to the basement, got on the computer, and started making some phone calls. I was convinced that there had to be some way to get money to afford this. So, I called the Canadian Cancer Society, and I spoke with them about the idea of funding my trips. It was a mess. They offered me $25 a week — and that was in Canadian funds. I was supposed to live on that when I went to the States! Great. That would get me a Happy Meal and a tent parked on the side of the road. I couldn't believe $25 was all they could offer. I kept thinking, all these people raise money for the Canadian Cancer Society, for what? The truth is, there's a lot of bureaucracy and red tape involved. The majority of the money raised goes towards research, not necessarily individual cases.

Then, I called the Canadian Breast Cancer Foundation and spoke with one of the higher officials. He wasn't able to help at all. I started to get really angry, and I gave him a piece of my mind.

And then he put me on hold. I was so angry at this point, and even more so that I had been cut off. When he came back on the line, I was beginning to think I had a chance. And then he told me to wait until the drug was offered in Canada.

"I don't have a *cold*," I told him, outraged. "I have *cancer*. I can't wait! I don't have *time* to wait! No!"

I hung up the phone, feeling totally discouraged. Sitting there, wracking my brain about what to do next, I was startled by the phone ringing.

"Hello," an Englishman said, asking for me.

"Yes?"

"You don't know me, but my name is Ray Matthey. I heard about your situation. I'd like to help you."

A social worker from Ottawa General Hospital had phoned Ray up, informing him of my situation. He wasn't sure what he could do, but he took my number and called me up.

An ex-air force vet, Mr. Matthey had also worked for Bell Canada before retiring. His daughter, Jeannette, once a radio journalist for CBC, had died of breast cancer at age 37, and a year after, his wife Sue Saunders passed away from the same disease. Before Sue's death, they created a cancer foundation out of their personal estate. Thus, with

$198,000 in the account, the Saunders–Matthey Foundation was born.

The first objective of the Saunders–Matthey Foundation is to put themselves out of business: namely, support finding a cure to end this disease. The way to do that is through the second objective: finding the causes, and progressively eliminating them through improved detection procedures. Also, the foundation believes in improved treatments combining both traditional methods with natural and spiritual therapies that focus on the individual needs of the patient. Believing that independent, unbiased research by the governmental health agencies regarding the effectiveness of natural health products could lead to new possibilities, the foundation essentially wants to explore all options.

While women have all the same component parts, both on the exterior and interior, each has a unique genetic makeup, which is why the "magic bullet" approach seems simplified. He believed if he was able to help one person have a renewed hope for a future, even if there was no guarantee that the Herceptin would be a success in my case, that just the chance to try was payoff enough. The fact that he could provide that hope for me gave him a sense of purpose.

It was like I had just met Santa Claus. He took me under his wing.

"You deal with your father, and whatever you need to do right now. I don't want you to have to worry about absolutely anything. We're going to take care of everything for you."

"Oh . . . my . . . God," I whispered. I had goosebumps. I know now that if it hadn't been for this man, I would never have had a chance to recover.

I went over to Mr. Matthey's home for supper with Tante Denise. The house, in Kanata, Ontario, was beautiful. He even *looked* like Santa Claus to me. An elderly man with a trimmed white moustache and beard, he had an elegance to him. It was an emotional evening for both of us. For Mr. Matthey, the situation brought his daughter to mind. Unable to help her, he saw the opportunity to help me, a woman of roughly the same age. That night, as we spoke, I had visions of what I could do in order to give back the money he would be using to support me.

"I could run across Canada!" I said excitedly, visions of Terry Fox in my head. "Actually, I could *rollerblade* across Canada! We can raise all this money, and I can give it back to you!"

I wanted to do anything I could.

"No," he said kindly. "You don't have to do anything. You need your energy. You need to build up your strength."

As Texas was really too far, I managed to get my treatments moved to New Haven, Connecticut at the Yale–New Haven Hospital where a research program on Herceptin had been established. The Saunders–Matthey Foundation paid the hotel bill directly, as well as the Yale–New Haven Hospital fees. Any other travel costs would be paid back upon receiving the receipts. The treatments in New Haven would cost $550 Canadian per trip. While there, they would measure my progress, along with the progress of the other test patients, to determine how effective Herceptin was. My first treatment was scheduled for August 28 — only a few weeks away.

"Even if it doesn't work," Mr. Matthey told me, "You are making a positive contribution." But the fact that I was getting this opportunity at all gave me hope.

I knew this could be my chance for life, but I still had to take things one day at a time.

CHAPTER SEVEN

Final Good-Byes

It was a beautiful summer day when we left for New Haven, Connecticut, and yet, it was a very sad scene. Tante Denise and Oncle Fern were driving me down in their motor home. My parents, who so desperately wanted to come with us, had decided at the last minute not to join us. Dad was quite sick at this point, and didn't want to take any chances, especially crossing the border into the States with no health coverage. So, it would be just the three of us. We left at around 10 in the morning, with both my parents standing in the driveway, seeing us off. My mother looked so lost, while my father appeared sad and worried, like a little boy.

I wasn't doing too well health-wise, either. By the time the motor home had turned the first corner, I was asleep. I slept for most of the trip down. We had a nice lunch at a restaurant called Lulu's half-way there, but all three of us were preoccupied with thoughts of my father. As we continued on our journey, I watched the landscape whiz by, not feeling particularly good about anything. The trees were so nice and green and everything was blooming. It was as though life was just beginning.

We arrived in New Haven at about 12 at night, exhausted and anxious about the following day. There was no foreseeable reason why anything should go wrong. When we arrived at the Yale–New Haven

Hospital the next day, however, things didn't run as smoothly as we had hoped.

Tante Denise and I were sitting in a little room, giggling and laughing at everything, waiting for the doctors to come. I don't know if it was stress, nerves, or both, but we couldn't stop. Here I was, sick, and supposed to try a new treatment that we weren't sure would actually work, and yet I was having a great time. I knew, somehow, that it was going to be okay.

"You're going to make me pee in my pants! Stop it!" Denise howled at me.

Finally, we discovered what was taking the doctors so long to arrive. I didn't have cancer.

"What?!" I asked incredulously.

The chart they had, for some reason, showed no signs of the illness. They didn't have my X-rays or the results of my Her-2/neu test, and so therefore I couldn't have the Herceptin treatment.

"Listen," I said to the nurse, slowly. "I didn't drive all this way — *eight* hours — for you to tell me I don't have cancer when *two weeks* ago, they were telling me I was dying."

"You'll need to go back and get your results, because we need to be sure you have the right cancer," she told me.

"Do you have any idea how far I've come?" I asked, calmly. "I've got a better idea for you. Why don't you call Dr. Young at the Ottawa Hospital and have it couriered here? I will take the weekend off, and I'll be back here on Monday. You'll have the results and you'll know that I have cancer. And then, I can have my treatment. Okay?"

"Okay," she said.

So they made a few calls, and discovered that yes, it was fine to courier the information so that I wouldn't have to drive another 16 hours retrieving the charts. So, Monday, August 31, should the hospital be satisfied with the results, I would have my first Herceptin treatment.

I believe everything happens for a reason. In this case, taking that weekend and spending time with my family was just what the doctor ordered — treatment for my emotional, spiritual self.

We had a whole weekend ahead of us, so my uncle, aunt, and I decided, let's make the best of this. My cousin Marc, his wife Olga, and his two young daughters Emillie and Sophie, had planned on coming to New Haven to support me through my treatment. They were camping in Rhode Island, which wasn't too far away. So instead of them coming to us, we decided to join them.

We drove out to see them, and once there, we parked the motor home and relaxed. We made up some Caesars, then took our chairs and sat on the beach by the ocean. A nice-looking man came by, and started talking to Oncle Fern.

"That's my niece," he explained. "We're down here because she has cancer and she's going to have this new treatment." He started telling this man the whole story, and after he left, I turned to Fern.

"Mon Oncle," I said teasingly. "How am I going to meet someone if you keep telling them I've got cancer?!"

"Oh," he said. "Oh, I did that, didn't I?"

We laughed, the Caesars starting to make us feel really good. So, we headed back to the trailer and made another one. We drank two Caesars each, and they went straight to our heads. I think it was due to all the stress we had left at home, plus the hospital fiasco.

My aunt and I went to phone my dad still dressed in our bathing suits. Both of us were giggling uncontrollably. My father could hear me laughing in the background as he spoke with Denise. He was so worried about us, thinking we had been drinking because we had received bad news, and therefore couldn't have my treatment.

"What's wrong with her?" he asked Denise, concerned.

"She's just had too many Caesars," she said. "She's okay."

We spent the next day with Marc, Olga, and the girls on the beach, swimming in the ocean. There was a large outdoor shower to rinse off in, so we all piled in and got our picture taken. It was a day filled with unconditional love, which I needed desperately. I bonded with those two little girls right away. Emillie and Sophie became my Disney babies. I had very little hair at this point, but they would touch my head and say:

"Ma Tante Sue, you're so pretty."

They told me they would pray at night for me before they went to bed. At meals, they would both have to sit next to me, putting their plates beside mine. Their love was just what I was looking for. When I was with Steph, I hadn't seen them as often. After my marriage fell apart, however, I realized just how important my family and the people I love are to me. I had been feeling lost, and there they were, these two beautiful children, giving me those hugs that I needed.

We had a lovely weekend, returning to New Haven on Sunday night. After asking for directions, and continuing our search, we gave up looking for the Sleeping Giant campsite where we had planned on staying. Oncle Fern, who was 6'2", inherited the nickname instead, and we parked in a rest area and slept in the motor home for the night.

The following day, I went in for my first treatment. For over 90 minutes, I was administered Herceptin (rhuMAb HER2) intravenously through my portocath. It was three times the amount that I receive now. The hope was that the Herceptin would prevent further tumour growth, possibly even decreasing the size of the present one. Or, it would have little to no effect. I would have it administered once a month at the Yale–New Haven hospital, and would be subjected to other tests for research purposes. Then, for the three weeks in between, I would go once a week to Ottawa General and have a half-hour Herceptin treatment there.

When my time was up, we all hustled back into the motor home. I felt feverish and had back pains due to the first dose. I tried to rest while my aunt and uncle booted towards the border, trying to get me home as fast as they could. I couldn't get any health insurance for the U.S. because of my cancer, and the last thing we needed were expensive medical bills. After a couple of hours of driving, my fever went down, and I started to feel a bit better.

Summer had brought life, a new venture, a new treatment, and a new start for me. September brought the changing leaves. It was as though death was setting in . . . and that was what was happening with my father. The trees were starting to become skeletons, as was my father. My second journey to New Haven was just as bittersweet. While it felt good to get away, it was difficult to leave because my father was getting worse. We didn't know what would happen while we were gone.

While Oncle Fern came with us one more time, most of the journeys to New Haven were with Tante Denise, driving in my father's van. My aunt and I would drive down to New Haven, sleep in the hotel next to the hospital, I would have my treatment the next day, then we would leave straight away. We would stop in New Hampshire in the evening at a hotel. Then, after dinner, we would relax in the pool and hot tub, and finish the drive early the next morning.

My trips to New Haven were my chance to have a mini-break from what was happening at home. It let me live a little, even if I was going down for treatment. I felt like a normal person during those trips. My mother, however, wasn't given the chance to take a break. She was living in a personal hell every day, while my father's health was deteriorating rapidly.

Often, I would have to take his oxygen mask off in order to administer his asthmatic pump, which helped him breathe by expanding his lungs. I would joke with him, stealing his mask, and breathing in the oxygen pretending I was in one of those spas in California.

"Hey!" I would say in an American accent, "Good oxygen, Dad! This is pretty cool!"

My father would smile, pumping his inhaler, lying there amid his pink sheets.

One of Dad's favourite places to go to was the casino in Ottawa. My cousin Manon and I decided one day to make a special trip with him, even though he was having difficulties breathing. He loved the slot machines. After our trip to the casino, we decided to go out for supper at the Ritz. We ordered, and started to eat, but my dad couldn't even finish his meal.

"You girls finish," he told us. Our van was parked outside, so he went out to it, and lay down in the back. We abandoned our meals and took him straight home. He slept the entire way. Manon and I stayed quiet for the whole ride, both of us knowing that Dad didn't have much more time with us.

That was the last big event of his life.

After a couple of phone conversations, I started seeing Steph secretly. He was working hard at trying to make things better for me. On my birthday, I went out for dinner with my cousins, then left early to head over to Steph's. When I got there, I found a ring, a matching necklace, and a birthday card. It was what I needed at the time — comfort, attention, and love.

My father was sleeping in a hospital bed at this point, with the bars up at the sides. I would sit at the end of his bed, singing to him, just being close by. We also had a chart on the wall listing all the times and dates for medicinal purposes. His medication had gotten really complicated at this point. While we had a nurse there almost 24 hours a day, there were things we had to learn — how to give him his asthmatic pump, how to adjust the oxygen levels, how to give him his morphine, how to take him to the washroom, as well as recording what and when he ate. I had made up a chart on cardboard, and the final date written down was October 11. Instead of making a whole new chart, I just flipped it over a couple of days early. I figured it was only two days, and we needed a longer-term chart because the meds were getting mixed up. So, I said I'd continue the chart on the back.

My Dad knew he was leaving us at this point, and had asked to speak to everyone individually on the Saturday. When it was my turn, I went in to see him, took his hand, and listened carefully. I knew he was going somewhere with this.

"You weren't okay with this at the beginning," he said. "You didn't want to accept this. But now . . . now I think you're okay with it."

He made me promise to be good to my mother, because in my life, I had always been closer to him, and taken his side. Now that he was leaving, he wouldn't be able to keep the peace. He mentioned this because tensions were running high in the house, and Mom and I had had a few arguments. I had to learn to compromise.

That day, my Dad went through everyone. At the end, he asked for a particular photograph: his wedding photo. Black and white, it is a beautiful 8 x 10 picture of my parents from their wedding album. I went *crazy* trying to find this picture.

"MOM! WE NEED TO GET HIM A PICTURE! WHERE IS THE PICTURE?!"

Once we found it, my father took it in his hands and said:

"There's my beautiful wife."

He held it, and then slowly drifted off to sleep. Taking the picture from him, we placed it nearby so he could see it.

That night, October 10th, was my high school's 25-year reunion, and Steph asked me if I wanted to go with him for supper, then attend the event. His sister would also be coming up from New York to join us. So, I got ready, then headed into my father's room to help him make a trip to the washroom. As I was holding him, I noticed his physical stature once more.

"Jeez, Dad, look at your stomach. You're so skinny. God, I wish I was like that."

He looked right at me, then suddenly burst out crying. Then, he started hugging me tight, while I kept trying to hold him up.

"I hope you won't ever be like this," he said quietly.

I felt the tears coming right there. Once he was finished, I helped him back into bed.

"Will I see you tomorrow?" he asked.

"Of course! Of course!" I told him.

"Where are you going?"

"I'm going to my high school reunion with Steph and his sister," I said.

"Okay," he said. "Have fun, be careful."

That night, I went to my reunion, staring at everyone, everything feeling surreal. That night, I didn't want to go back to the house where my father was. I slept at Steph's instead. At eight the next morning, I bolted out of bed.

"I've got to get home I've got to get home," I said over and over.

I knew there was something wrong. As soon as I walked in the house, into my father's room, I knew. It was time. I hadn't eaten much the night before, and I had skipped breakfast. My mother's brother, Oncle Jean-Guy, tried to make me eat a sandwich, but it sat alone on the table. I didn't want to eat. Instead, I went back to my father's room to be with him; I knew how precious time was at this point.

My father had started making gurgling noises, his body jumping slightly. The nurse had explained to us what was going to happen. So, I called Oncle Jean-Guy and told him to locate everybody. Then I called Fern and Denise. They had finally taken a couple of days to relax after all this stress, and suddenly, they needed to rush back.

"He's leaving," I told them.

In my room, I had a stereo. I put on a Frank Sinatra CD, just for Dad. Suddenly, "My Way" was filtering through the house.

"*And now, the end is near, and so I face, the final curtain. . . .*"

My father needed to use the washroom, so I helped him out. We both stared in shock as his urine came out. It was black.

"Oh damn oh damn . . ." was all he could say.

"Don't be saying that now!" I told him, "We're going to have to do a whole rosary!"

The whole family had arrived to be by his side — everyone except my grandmother in Quebec. She was 87 years old, with a heart problem, and we didn't want her to have to go through this. We all held his hand, standing around him, waiting. I went into the other room for a short time, completely exhausted, and lay down on the bed.

Ten minutes before my Dad passed away, they called me back into the room. I slipped my arm underneath his head, and sang him the song that he always used to sing to me when I was a little girl.

"I want to live my life to the fullest. I never want to imprison it. If I feel like throwing my hands in the air, just let me, 'cause that's what I want to do. Let me live my life and be happy." My Dad would always say that song reminded him of me, his little black sheep.

I took his hand in mine, because I wanted to touch it. Soon, I wouldn't be feeling the warmth anymore, and it would grow cold. He was surrounded by brothers, sisters, nieces, nephews, even two priests — Père Vaillancourt and Père Dumoulin — friends of his. He was a loved man.

As my father slipped away, mon Oncle Fern decided he had said his good-byes, and that it was time for him to go home. The motor home was in the driveway, and I watched it as it drove around the corner. At that moment, my Dad died. We tried to call Fern back, but it was too late. Everything felt so strange at that moment.

I recalled how, the day before, Tante Denise and I had been talking in the bedroom about my Dad, and he stopped us.

"Hey!" he said, "I'm not gone yet! The motor home is parked in the driveway, but it's not gone yet."

"Who's driving?" ma tante asked.

"Jesus," he told us.

It could easily be blamed on the morphine, but I sensed it was something different. He was right. The motor home left the driveway, and my Dad died right then. I felt the warmth drain away from his hand and his fingers grow stiff.

We all left the room, and the nurses took over. First they repositioned his body before it grew stiff. Then, they wrapped a light pink towel around his jaw and head, tying a knot at the top. When I saw it, I couldn't understand why they would do that. They told me it was in order to keep his jaw shut. I was always terrified of dead bodies, but when I went into that room, I could actually hug him. He was the first dead person whom I was able to touch.

I returned to the living room, and watched as a car pulled into the driveway, and a man in a black suit got out. They had come for his body. Mission stood there, silent. Normally, he would bark at someone who approached the door, but he just sat there. He appeared lost, sensing something was wrong. I went into my room, lying on my bed and weeping. I didn't want to watch them roll my Dad away. As far as I was concerned, he had already left.

My whole family was there to support me, and yet I felt alone. Life is so precious and every loss feels different. Sylvie knew I was seeing Steph, and how important it would be for me to have him there. She called him up so he could come and be with me. He understood how hard this was for me, because he knew how close I was with my Dad. He came, even though it was difficult for him, and was very supportive. My whole family was aware of what had happened between us, and were not happy with him. And yet, he came for me because he did care, in his own way. That night, he slept over, staying by my side.

Oncle Fern was the one who discovered the cardboard I had flipped. The final date on the first side was October 11, Thanksgiving

Sunday. The day he finally left us. We puzzled over why it had ended on that specific date. He had promised my mother that he would not pass away on her birthday, October 14, and he'd kept his promise. His funeral, however, was another matter.

His funeral was held at the Boulerice Funeral Home. Denise, Fern, and I were the ones who did all the arrangements. Because it was fall, we chose some beautiful fall-coloured roses to drape on the casket, next to a photograph of him and me at Mt. Tremblant. There was a line of people outside the funeral home, all there to pay their final respects to my Dad. Old friends of mine came, along with some ex-boyfriends. Little Marco showed up with a Coke bottle filled with roses, just for Dad. It was lovely to see all the people there. I was amazed at how many showed up.

The funeral was held on my mother's and my Grandmother Giroux's birthday. I sat with my mother in the church for the service, and the priest wished my mother and grandmother a happy birthday. There were tons of priests at the service, all friends of my father. He had spent time getting to know them at all the spiritual weekend retreats he had attended. The church was just as packed. As the priest gave the eulogy, I was lost in a different world. It felt so weird to be in that church for my father's funeral: the same church I had gone to every Sunday with my parents. I found myself drifting back in time, remembering all those moments we had spent in the church: my first Communion, singing in the choir, with my parents watching me, proud of their little girl. When I would sit with them, I always wanted the aisle seat, but that was Dad's. So, I sat between them.

Now, it was only my mom and I, and I sat in the aisle. As much as I believed Dad was right beside me, I still felt alone. I wanted to hold him, to touch him, to feel the warmth of his body.

My father was cremated, with a memorial placed on a stone wall in a small cemetery just outside of Cornwall. We all have problems that can end up consuming us, then you go to the cemetery and realize just how little we are. Every tombstone has a story. If only we knew what was waiting for us on the other side, things would be totally different. I look at the ocean, at the sky, and can't see any end. That's where my father is. Everywhere.

After my father's funeral, I moved back in with Steph, once more hoping we could make things right. I could feel the Herceptin working, which made me all the more grateful for Ray Matthey's support. Ray never got the chance to meet my father, but he did come to the funeral. I wanted to give something back to his foundation, and to distract myself from the hurt of losing my dad. So, I put a committee together, and arranged for our first meeting to be at the Parkway. That night, I nominated my cousin Marc for the position of chairman, which he accepted. Sylvie became the secretary. About thirty people were in that room, and I was amazed by the amount of support. Olga and Manon, my cousins Barb and Charlene, my cousins Nicole and Marie, and Mary Bard was there along with her friend Claire. My nurse, Roseanne, and her daughter came to support us, and even Adele Bray from the Boulerice Funeral Home showed up.

The plan was to raise money that would go towards the expenses from my treatments. We called it "A Chance for Life."

Mary and Claire came up with the idea for a wine and cheese. They took over, doing the majority of organization while the rest of us did what was necessary. We set the date for December, giving us a short time to prepare. That meant getting on the ball — finding a venue, distributing tickets, getting donations, and also creating literature explaining what the event was for. We got to it right away.

The venue we chose was the Weave Shed in Cornwall. It was an old renovated cotton mill with hardwood floors, sitting right on the water. Lisa Caneb, whose family owned the building, helped out significantly. They had created offices in the building, along with a theatre for small productions. Whenever there was a show, she put aside one dollar from each ticket in order to support the event. In the end, the money raised paid the expense for renting the hall. I was so grateful for all the help. Everyone was so generous when it came to supporting the event. The problem was, while the arrangements were going so well, I was still mourning the death of my father.

I still had my monthly Herceptin treatments in New Haven, although with the change in season, they grew more bleak. Marc's wife, Olga, came with me on my November 19th trip to New Haven. Olga's mother had died of breast cancer, and while I was losing my father, we became much closer. She, too, was an only child. The whole trip involved a lot of sharing. One night, we had a lovely supper out, then went to bed. When I woke up, I realized I was tightly hugging Olga. I apologized, wondering why she hadn't just woken me up. Olga told me it was cute, then later told Marc she didn't dare move!

The Chance for Life benefit was approaching fast. I was still grieving for my father, which made it tough. Steph was responsible for selling most of the tickets to the wine and cheese. One night, while he was at another fundraising event, he started selling tickets like crazy, and called to tell me about it. I could hear the excitement in his voice. That was what made our relationship confusing: good one minute, tough the next.

The date finally arrived, and was quite successful for six to seven weeks of preparation. While it was not a black tie event, it was still very glamorous. An event like that worked well in Cornwall, simply because there aren't too many like it that require people to get all dressed up. We had a jazz trio playing, and had a variety of wines and cheeses, all donated. The mayor of Cornwall, along with our MP and MPP showed up, and of course, Ray Matthey was there. I was asked to speak, and I talked of my father, and the gift of being given a second chance.

While the event ended quite early — 11 or 12 — people stayed from start to finish, which was unexpected. Considering how rushed we were to put it together, we didn't know how much we would raise, but we ended up with $2200! Mr. Matthey was very pleased with the results, considering we had pulled everything together on such short notice. The community support was exceptional.

It was just before Christmas when I got the news I had been waiting for. The CT scan results showed that my lymph nodes had not only stopped growing, but had actually *shrunk*! I was feeling human again, and it was all due to Herceptin. I had no more difficulties with side effects, and my hair was slowly growing back. It was giving me life, and taking it was as simple as drinking a glass of water. And yet, while the medication was helping, there was more healing that needed to be done. My eating habits had to change, along with eradicating all the negative influences in my life.

My cousin Marc would always say "God has a plan for everyone — we just haven't figured out what His plan is for you yet, Sue."

It was time to find out.

CHAPTER EIGHT

A Change for Life

Ray Matthey started to make inquiries with CTV about doing a short feature on me, hoping that it would promote the Saunders–Matthey Foundation and show breast cancer patients that there were other options. Dianne Duffy from CBC caught the short segment, and contacted the Foundation. They, in turn, put her in touch with me. So, as Christmas approached, I was interviewed by Dianne Duffy. I had a great time doing it. Unfortunately, the Herceptin trials were over, and the treatments would only be available in the U.S.

Hoffmann La Roche, the pharmaceutical company, was now working in partnership with Genentech, Inc. The Herceptin trials were almost over, meaning that the drug would now have to be paid for. Hoffmann La Roche, however, was working on a Canadian compassionate release program, which would be active in January 1999. I was so fortunate. If they hadn't done that, I would have been lost. Imagine, finally finding a treatment, only to have it taken away from you.

The show included an interview with another woman, one who was not fortunate enough to be receiving Herceptin. Her interview, in contrast to mine, sparked a few people to start writing to the government, hoping to get the drug approved in Canada faster than it would normally take. In January and February, I got on the letter writing bandwagon.

Honourable Mike Harris.

Dear Premier:

As a breast cancer patient in Ontario currently taking Herceptin, the breakthrough drug for breast cancer, I am writing to ask for your help to make Herceptin available to breast cancer patients in Ontario. And I am willing to help you make this happen. What makes Herceptin so unique and truly breakthrough? Herceptin is the first new therapy for breast cancer since Taxol in 1994. Unlike chemotherapy, which attacks your entire body to destroy the cancer, Herceptin is a "smart drug" which attacks cancer at the gene level. Herceptin identifies, selects, and blocks a protein found on the surface of some breast cancer cells known as HER2. Excess amounts of HER2 lead to uncontrolled growth characteristics of cancer. Approximately 25–30 per cent of women with breast cancer produce too much HER2, making them candidates for Herceptin therapy.

Herceptin offers hope to patients like myself, who failed on chemotherapy and who until now, had no treatment options. Treatment with Herceptin has resulted in higher one-year survival rates among women with metastatic breast cancer. Recently, CBC Newsworld did a story about me and what I was going through to get access to Herceptin. Until I was able to get Herceptin in Canada, I drove 8 hours to New Haven, Connecticut, from my home in Cornwall, once a month to get treatment. Now I am able to get Herceptin at the Ottawa Regional Cancer Centre through a clinical trial.

*I have seen you on the news talking about your gov-
ernment's concern for Ontario's health care system and
the patients who use it. That is why I am turning to you
to have Ontario lead the way in breast cancer treatment.*

I wanted him to support the federal government getting Herceptin
approved before the fall of 1999, which was the projected date. At that
point, the only access to Herceptin in Canada was through Hoffmann
La Roche's special access program, and Canada would have to go
through their own clinical trials. I also felt that Herceptin should be
available through Cancer Care Ontario. I explained that while it was
expensive on a "per patient" basis, the only eligible women were the
ones who produce too much HER2. It wasn't a cure, I admitted that,
but it did give women a chance to fight.

I wrote similar letters to Joe Fontana, our MP, and the Hon. Paul
Martin, the Minister of Finance. The Saunders–Matthey Foundation
also got on the bandwagon, writing to Alan Rock, the Health Minister
for Health Canada, also encouraging an early acceptance of Herceptin.
While a response to these was important to me, there was another
letter from which I was hoping for a response. I had just read the book
*Her2: The Making of Herceptin, a Revolutionary Treatment for Breast
Cancer* by Robert Bazell. I had wanted to learn more about the drug I
was taking. When I found out that Genentech, Inc. was the company
that was producing it, I felt compelled to write them a letter. I wanted
to tell them how great it was to have a company coming up with something new, something other than chemo. I also told them that if they
needed me, I would love to represent them in some way.

I got a lovely response from Judith Heyboer, the Senior VP of Human
Resources at Genentech, thanking me for my story and for sharing it
with them. She passed on my letter to the corporate communications
department, extending her hopes that they could keep me in mind as

a spokesperson. I then received a phone call out of the blue, from a man at Genentech. I was totally shocked. He was very kind, and told me how much he appreciated the letter, but explained there wasn't much he could do for me in the way of work. He suggested I call Hoffmann La Roche.

After my CBC interview, I spoke with Helen Stone at Hoffmann La Roche, who invited me to lunch. On January 20, I had my treatment in Ottawa, then met up with her. We quickly became friends, enjoying each other's company, and she suggested I come to Hoffmann La Roche in Ottawa and tell my story. Hoffmann La Roche hadn't had much contact with the patients who had been on the drug, so this was a nice opportunity to change that.

The first time I spoke at Hoffmann La Roche was in Toronto. There was an inter-company lunch, giving employees the chance to attend different educational sessions. I spoke with the employees, telling them my story. I had had my last treatment in New Haven on February 4, so now, due to Hoffmann La Roche's generosity in keeping me on the compassionate release program in Canada, I was having all my weekly sessions in Ottawa.

I spoke of my experiences and fears about chemotherapy, and the problems I had had with infections. I told them how, while in New Haven, the doctors wanted me to have chemo in conjunction with the Herceptin as a part of the study, but that I flat-out refused. I explained that the commute once a week was not an issue, and that I treated it as a holiday. The fact was, I had taken a whole slew of poisons, and nothing would stop the cancer. After taking Herceptin for only a few months, my lymph nodes had shrunk. "Essentially," I explained, "It changed my life. It *saved* my life."

While I was growing more interested in working with Hoffmann La Roche and becoming more active in breast cancer awareness, my marriage was once again falling apart. Steph and I went away to

Florida in early March, but the tensions were growing. Once back, I started speaking with my cousin Sylvie about it.

"I can't do this," I told her, "It's back to the same thing."

I kept looking at our marriage and thinking 'Is this why I cried so much? Is this why I tried to kill myself? To come back to *this*? What for?' It had become a marriage of convenience.

At the end of March, I went to Hamilton with Ray Matthey for an environmental conference. I called home the entire five days I was there, but Steph never answered. I was worried about Mission. I was also realizing that I wasn't getting the support I needed. It was time to start thinking about what it was I really wanted.

While I was at the conference, I had the opportunity to listen to Samuel Epstein, a speaker on environmental issues. I was so intrigued when he was talking that I went and bought his book. Afterwards, I had the chance to speak with him. I asked him all about asbestos and about my father. After a brief chat with him, an idea came into my head. I wondered that while my father had been exposed to asbestos, had it affected my mother somehow when she was pregnant, thus instigating the cancer? It was a question I have never been able to answer. Then, I started thinking about my father, and the environment he'd been exposed to, and once again wondered why I was living in such a negative one myself.

Ray and I drove back from Hamilton, talking all the way. It was then that he became a surrogate father for me, someone to confide in. We had a great conversation, and I started telling him about Steph. His point was simple: he couldn't tell me what I had to do, but if Steph wasn't there for me . . .

When I got to the house, Steph was there. I was feeling the exact same thing I felt as I stood alone in the airport after my trip to Seattle. Suddenly, I was wondering why it was we had gotten back together in the first place. I had been feeling so vulnerable during my father's illness, and Steph had been there. But moving back in the day after my father died? I should have known better.

A few weeks later, I was sitting downstairs in the tub. After I lit some candles and sank into the water, I felt the tears come. So, I began praying to my father. Every time I prayed to him, I felt as though he was right beside me.

"Dad," I said quietly, "You have to do something drastic for me to leave him because you know I won't. I'm going to put up with him, stay with him otherwise. This is not the life I want to live." I was on my treatment and was getting better, but I still felt as though I was in a rush for time. I wanted to live life to the fullest every minute of every day, not in fear.

So I prayed to my dad as I prepared to head out to our friend Chris and Julie's place for a barbecue. I called Steph at work earlier to ask him if he wanted to go. He agreed. I picked up a couple of steaks and some wine for the evening.

"Something drastic, Dad," I prayed quietly, "Either it works out and makes me happy, or he has to do something wickedly wrong to make me open my eyes and leave for good."

That night we went to the barbecue, and while outwardly things appeared okay between us, I was feeling bitter. The relationship just wasn't there. We returned home, and I went upstairs and called Joanne in Vancouver. We started discussing the idea of going on a trip down south. She had a pamphlet that offered access to a sailboat and a crew, and the idea was quite exciting. I hung up the phone and returned to the kitchen, to find Steph sitting at the counter.

"What are you doing?" I asked him.

He was reading my medical file.

Every time I had to go to New Haven, I had to bring my entire medical life with me. The doctors needed all the information, so I kept it at the house. In the file there was a piece where one of the doctors had noted his concern that physical abuse was a factor in my life due to bruises he had seen on my arm. Steph grew angry at this, accusing me of telling people bad things about him. The fight grew and finally, I lost it.

"GET OUT!" I screamed.

When I got angry like that, it set Steph off. He hit me. I fell to the ground and the next thing I knew, he was beating the side of my face onto the ceramic tiled floor. I passed out, and came around with Mission licking my face. There was no immediate sign of Steph. Terrified, I rushed upstairs and hid in the bathroom with my foot against the door. Time became so warped . . . I have no idea how long I stood there like that. Finally, I found the guts to run into my bedroom, grab the phone, and run back to the bathroom, where I dialled 911. Then, I called Sylvie.

You don't call 911 unless you really need to. Suddenly, fire trucks, an ambulance, and police cars were arriving. It felt like the whole world had just shown up at my door. I was petrified, hearing them come through the front door. An officer started trying to coax me out of the washroom, convincing me that I would be okay. I was still afraid Steph was in the house. All I could think was, I don't want to get hit again, get screamed at again. It was as though it was a movie that you want to switch off, but can't.

Finally I got out of the bathroom and made the cops search the entire house, looking under the beds and checking all the closets. I even made them check downstairs behind one of our mirrors! My cousin Sylvie showed up, as did my friends Chris and Julie.

"What difference does it make if he's here?" they asked me. "You're not sleeping here. You're coming with us."

All I wanted was for everything to stop. My face was all black and blue on one side. I let myself cry, with Julie and Sylvie guiding me to the door. Just before we left the house, the phone rang.

"It's him it's him!" I whimpered.

Sgt. Murphy, the female officer, answered the phone. Steph started yelling on the other end, believing it to be me.

"Stephane," she said calmly, "This is Sgt. Murphy. Either you can make it easy on yourself and go to the police station, or we're going to pick you up. Based on the call display, we know you're calling from your office."

All of a sudden, the voice on the other end grew quiet. I never found out what happened to him that night, or how he was bailed out. I went to the hospital with Julie and Sylvie, getting checked out for a concussion. That night, I crashed at Julie's home. The first time I left Steph, it was April 18, 1998. The second, and final, was April 20, 1999.

The next day I called my lawyer. I didn't have a clue about what to do, and on top of all that, it was a Wednesday. I had to drive to Ottawa for my treatment. I wasn't looking forward to facing Dr. Young with my face all bruised. As I sat there, alone in the treatment room, one nurse started crying with me. It was like a soap opera. Here I was, having my cancer treatment after my husband had beaten me. Every time I would go to treatments, I would see loving families around the patient, supporting them. It was making me feel like a victim. I kept asking myself, why is this happening to me? The only solace I had was the belief that everything happens for a reason. I just wanted to understand the reason.

I returned to the house in Cornwall, and had the locks in the house changed immediately. A restraining order had been issued on Steph, preventing him from coming near the house. We stopped speaking to each other entirely for around nine months. I had forgotten about him, and had finally seen why I should not be with him.

I started taking a Dale Carnegie course in Ottawa on public speaking. The decision had been made; I knew what I wanted to do with my life. I wanted to be a public speaker. The courses were held every

Wednesday night, so I would arrange for the latest possible appointment at the hospital for my treatment, then head to class afterwards.

I still missed my father terribly, but my spirits were high. As the summer came, I found my self-confidence growing and my life stabilizing. I continued working for Dr. Leboeuf and continued my treatments — my life felt like my own again. Spending time with my family was also a priority. My little niece, Emillie, came to stay with me briefly, which was a special treat. We went out to Dairy Queen for lunch, then shopped for hair products, with the final destination being my mother's swimming pool. I was explaining to her that it was still the beginning of summer, so the water might be cold. And out of the blue, she asks me:

"Is little Jesus taking care of mon Oncle Claude?"

"Of course," I told her. "He's being well taken care of and he has all his friends and family up there."

"Does mon Oncle Claude have new shoes?"

"Of course," I said, chuckling lightly, "He has beautiful new shoes. He's got the best of everything up there. Everything is very very nice."

"Oh," she said, looking up at me.

This little girl was four years old and as she was asking me these questions, I had tears running down my face. She was looking at me, wondering why, but smart enough to know I was missing my dad.

"Does mon Oncle Claude up there have a swimming pool? I betcha his water's hot up there, eh, cause everything's nice up there."

"Yep, that's right," I said, smiling.

She caught on real quick. Children really are amazing that way.

I was still feeling the ache from losing my father. We all were. Sylvie told me a story later how she had taken her young son, Jonathan, to see my father's memorial marker up on the wall. He looked up at the little box, saying "I kind of miss him."

"We all do, you know."

"Well," he said, "Why don't you just tell him to come out of the little box and we can spend some time with him?"

I wish we could.

I was going back and forth to Toronto quite often, speaking here and there for Hoffmann La Roche, Canada. I had an interview with the *National Post* on August 9, and they did a large spread on my story. I was beginning to feel more and more comfortable with my new goals. The *National Post* article came out on the 18th of August, just two days after my first meeting for the 1999 "Chance for Life" wine and cheese fund-raiser.

This time, we gave ourselves much more time to prepare, with the projected date for the event being October 23. We wanted to expand it, adding more entertainment, with a silent auction as well as a live auction. This meant a lot of leg work going out to get donations of all sorts. We kept the name "Chance for Life" to keep the connection, but while the first event was designed to support my journeys to New Haven, this one was designed to give back to the Saunders–Matthey foundation on a larger scale. This time, the brochure created would update my progress.

Hoffmann La Roche flew me down to Toronto just as the *National Post* article came out. They had planned a speaking engagement for me, one with a larger audience. As I made my way to the gate, I noticed the amount of businessmen waiting around, and sure enough, I sat next to one reading a newspaper.

He was reading my story.

He turned to me, clued in, and asked if I was the same person. We started talking, and he ended up giving me a ride to my hotel. At first, I mentioned that I wanted a job with Hoffmann La Roche, but then he mentioned the idea of motivational speaking on a larger scale. He faxed my hotel a whole list of contacts, and different speakers' bureaux to call. To this day, we still keep in touch.

The first time I had flown down to Toronto, Hoffmann La Roche had arranged for a limo to pick me up and drive me to the offices or different functions I was attending. I had grown friendly with the driver, and got to know him well. He would always make sure to have a little cold cappuccino for me in the back seat. After the *National Post* article came out, he asked for my autograph. That felt strange. I had been talking to a variety of people since I began this new journey, and I realized that everyone has a story. Everyone is connected to someone with cancer. I survived, okay, but how does that make me unique? I was lucky. I was starting to discover my destiny. Having cancer had almost been a gift for me, because I was learning how to help others. And that made me feel good.

One night, as I was driving back on Highway 138 after my Dale Carnegie course, I found myself praying to my dad once more. I was used to talking to him all of the time. There was a full moon that night, and mellow French music crooned out from the stereo as I spoke. I was explaining that I didn't understand why the situation with Steph happened. I had a CT scan coming up, and I was feeling nervous about the possible results. It is something I always worry about. My concern was that I would never be able to mend the rift between Steph and I. Someday, when I'm on my dying bed, I want to know that I can die in peace. I wouldn't be able to do that knowing that I was at war with someone I had loved. I wanted to talk to Steph, to tell him I was sorry for whatever I did, and to try to understand why he did what he did. If that couldn't happen, then at least we could make peace. I had not forgotten everything he had done, but I had found a way to forgive him. And strange as it seemed, Steph was still one of the people I wanted at my bedside when I was dying.

Soon afterwards, I received a phone call from a friend of Steph's, asking if he could stop by and pick up Steph's skis.

"Let me think about it," I told him, "Call me in a few minutes."

I called up Jodi Lyn to ask her opinion.

"Ah," she said, "Give him his skis. You know, the poor guy doesn't even have his winter boots."

That was what I had wanted to do, but I needed to hear it from her. As soon as I hung up, his friend phoned once more. So I agreed to let him come by and pick up the skis. I placed them just outside the door, and made myself look busy. He didn't even come into the house. I was nervous about having contact with someone I hadn't seen in a long time. He came by, and I asked him how Steph was, and then I left the house.

When I came back, I hopped into the tub and had a bubble bath. I started praying once more about the whole scenario, hoping that Steph and I could one day come to terms with things. Right then, the telephone rang.

It was Steph.

I asked him if I could just see him for a bit. And even though the restraining order was still in effect, he showed up. We both talked, crying, going over everything he had done and I had done. He started telling me how his life had changed so drastically. Everybody knew what had happened between us. You can't walk around a town with a population of 46,000 and keep a secret — especially if your face is black and blue. He had lost friends over our fight, and I felt bad for that. I forgave him, yet I hadn't forgotten what he had done to me. So, there were a lot of mixed emotions between us.

Another night, he came over and had supper with me. It was *almost* as though we were friends. We watched *The Story of Us* that night, a movie with Bruce Willis and Michelle Pfeiffer about a couple who must decide whether or not their marriage is worth saving. The two of us got very emotional, simply because our story didn't end like the film. I didn't stand in a parking lot, telling Steph I wanted to get back together. Her final words, however, were very true. There are some memories that you've created with someone that you just can't share with anyone else. And when it came to Steph and I, there was a lot of truth to that statement. Yet, our lives had moved on, and the fact was, both of us still had many wounds that needed to heal. We knew we could never be together again.

The second wine and cheese arrived, and we had gone all out. I had the help of two new people who were indispensable: Rick and John. Mary was of course very active with this one, as well as Barb and Charlene. We started having meetings at my house, now that I was separated. It felt like a whole bunch of friends just sitting together, hanging out, brainstorming, with Rick and John as the key players guiding us through.

We wanted this evening to be a glamorous event, as it had been before, but on a much grander scale. Once again, we used the Weave Shed, only this time we decorated it much more elaborately. A lovely ivy archway with white lilies stood by a couple of the tables, while spiralled around the pillars were balloons the colours of the Saunders–Matthey Foundation logo — pink, silver, and burgundy.

I was overwhelmed by the generosity of the Cornwall community. All the food and gifts were donated *plus* we had monetary donations that went toward purchasing all the wine. A wine-tasting table was set up, and we had a small cabaret for the entertainment. The show lineup was all Broadway material, done by adults and kids. It was fantastic. John was instrumental in organizing that. The silent auction provided us with gifts of all sorts, including baskets, books, paintings, clothing, certificates, and more. The Dallas Cowboys even came through for us, donating a signed team photograph!

It was a full house, even before we had people buying tickets at the door. Most importantly, the evening ran smoothly. In the end, thanks to everyone's help, we were able to give the Saunders–Matthey Foundation a cheque for $14,000. Ray Matthey was overwhelmed. He had been pleased with the success of the first event, because we had done it in such short notice. After the second one, however, he was blown away by everyone's generosity.

The organizing crew was exhausted. Not only had we been meeting all week, but we had spent all of Friday and Saturday together setting up for the event, then Sunday morning cleaning up afterwards. We all took a well deserved break after that.

My life had become quite different from what it had been a few months earlier. I was focused on detoxifying my system, as well as reading different motivational books. Mary Bard and Lisa Canan were instrumental in helping me shift my diet as well. Lisa took me out shopping, introducing health food to me, and I bought tofu for the first time. I had begun using visualization tapes, picturing the positive things and seeing my tumour shrinking inside me. I had difficulties with that. Praying to my father was my positive thinking technique. Jodi Lyn would joke with me about it.

"Don't forget the big guy," she would say. "He's the one making the decisions."

"Dad's sitting right beside him," I'd tell her. "He can pull some strings."

On November 17, while I was in for one of my treatments, I met Christian. Earlier, he had apparently spotted me and asked the nurses who I was. The nurses, whom I had come to know very well, had become like relatives, and took it upon themselves to play match-maker. They gave him my *National Post* story, then introduced us. I didn't think much of it at the time, as I was still focused on my Dale Carnegie course. The following week, when I arrived at the clinic, there was a card for me from him. Inside, he had written his phone number. So, I decided that I would take the risk, and phone. He was out, but I had a nice conversation with his mother for about 15 minutes. The next day he returned my call, and we spoke for two hours.

Christian had melanoma and was finishing his treatments. He was a pilot and aerospace engineer in Toronto who was very caring and sensitive. He understood those rough times I had been through, and we had lots of interests in common, but I wasn't sure I was ready for a relationship. I was still going through the healing process. We started seeing each other, taking long walks in the woods, and we spent Christmas together.

In the middle of March, we went away to Hawaii together for two weeks. One morning, before the sun rose, I was feeling energetic, so I put my running shoes on, planning on taking a jog along the beach as I listened to my walkman. Just as I finished my jog, the sun started to come up. I sat down on the beach, took a drink of my water, and started praying to my father. As I looked over the ocean, I found myself thinking of times when we would go to Florida together, and how much he enjoyed that. It was then, praying to my dad and just missing him a lot, that I noticed all these little sparkles, like diamonds, floating around me. I started trying to catch them, not knowing what they were. A lady walked past me, and smiled, but the little floating sparkles wouldn't go away. Suddenly, I said the first thing that came into my mind.

"Hi, Dad."

I felt his presence surrounding me. It happened a second time as I lay on the beach, listening to some Hawaiian music. I was working with a positive visualization technique, in conjunction with praying to my father, only this time it was dusk. Once more, all of a sudden, the little diamonds appeared. This time, however, they were only on one side of my body, whereas the first time they had completely surrounded me. I contemplated this for the longest time — why were they only on one side? Then I realized they were on the side my cancer was.

I tried to see them again, but could not. They appeared only in Maui. Later on, I spoke with a woman who lives in Hawaii, and I shared my experience. She explained that Maui was filled with gods, and is one of the most healing places on earth. She agreed with me: it was most definitely my father.

As lovely as Christian was, I just wasn't ready for a relationship. I had thrown all of myself into my new path. In April 2000, Ray Matthey put on a huge fundraising event in Ottawa in honour of his wife's life. Set in Ottawa at La Contessa, the Saunders–Matthey Foundation raised $8000 for the evening. They had terrific media sponsorship from the *Ottawa Sun* and The Bear, one of Ottawa's radio stations. I was at the table of honour with the mayor of Ottawa and our MP. Jodi Lyn was my date for the evening, and we were also joined by Rick. It would be the first time I would speak in front of such a large audience — over 400 people — and I was nervous. I started my story from where I met Mr. Matthey, and how he had changed my life by being there for me when others hadn't. I spoke of my father, and how he had died just to give me a second chance.

Standing there, tears rolling down my face, I received my first standing ovation. One gentleman was so moved, he presented the foundation with a cheque for $500 immediately afterwards.

There was an amazing multi-course meal planned, but I hardly got a chance to eat. Suddenly, I was talking with CBC, and CTV, and doing all sorts of interviews. Near the end of the evening, the music began to play. Dr. Verma, the oncologist at Ottawa General who had dealt with me after the chemo, was also sitting at our table. "I Will Survive" boomed out of the speakers, and Dr. Verma and I started cutting it up on the dance floor. He cheered me on as I whipped around, still riding on the euphoria from my speech.

I will survive.

In June 2000, my divorce from Steph went through. He was finally moving on, as was I. Part of the agreement meant I had to leave our house. I started hunting around for apartments, then once more questioned what I was doing. That was the first clue. I had been dating someone for a couple of months, and I thought I had finally found someone whom I could enjoy being with. Paul wasn't from Cornwall, which I liked. While he was sensitive and kind, he just wasn't ready for a relationship, which I understood. Between having to find a new home and dealing with Paul, I realized my next step.

It was a Sunday when I called Joanne.

"What do you think about me moving to B.C.?" I asked her.

At first, she told me she thought it was wonderful, but then the practicality of the situation kicked in.

"Do you want to do this? Think about it," she said.

I continued my preparations for moving. I even quit my job with Dr. Leboeuf. A week or so later, I called Joanne up, and told her I was coming out. I was leaving no matter what. The only thing was, I still had a bunch of CT scan results to go through with my doctors, which I was feeling nervous about.

"You can't be leaving," my boss at work said. "I don't think you'll do it."

"If my CT scan results are bad, then I'll just go to Europe and travel around. But if they're good, I'm going to B.C." I told him.

The results came back, and my decision was made.

"I'm going to B.C."

Telling the nurses at Ottawa General Hospital was tough. They had seen me through chemo, and watched me grow healthier with Herceptin. They had talked with me and joked with me each week as I paced around the treatment room with my IV in hand. They had become like sisters, setting me up on dates, telling my story, telling me theirs. Suzanne, Judy, and Rita were three of the nurses with whom I shared an intimate part of my life. When I told them of my decision, they hugged me, crying but pleased. I knew I would miss them terribly.

A new life. A new start. A clean slate. I packed everything up into a U-Haul and walked around the empty house that was haunted by so many memories. A whole mass of images flashed through my head quickly, all at once. The good times with Steph, being sick, my father and mother taking care of me. My dad and I talking outside. Steph and I alone. It was so fast. I remembered the first day that Mission and I moved in, when he sniffed around the house, getting used to the space. All the first days, and all the last. When I left, I didn't shed one tear.

My father was with me, keeping me strong. I hopped in the U-Haul, and drove to my mother's place. That night, I slept in my dad's room. I had a hard time falling asleep that night. His presence and the excitement of the move were keeping me up. The next morning, I returned to my old house under the guise that I had forgotten something. This time, when I walked through the house, there were no memories. I had said my good-byes.

I left the keys on the counter, and walked away.

Epilogue

When I was dying, I prayed to God for a second chance, and He gave me one. It took me a little while to figure out what my direction should be, but I'm making an effort. My goal is to motivate others, to give them hope, to push them to take risks. I've always dreamed of having a street . . . the Suzanne Giroux Drive, like the Terry Fox one in Ottawa. Only, I don't want it to be "in memory of." I want to live to see it.

I no longer need the white picket fence, just a friend whom I can love. Life sometimes feels as though it is rushing by, and you need to grasp at everything. The key thing I have found is to recognize it is precious, and enjoy the time you have with the people you care about. Life is a celebration, and fun is most certainly allowed. It could be giggling uncontrollably during a car trip, or camping, or spending quiet time. So long as it's fun.

I have been saved by many different doctors, but the most important thing I realized is that they are just as human as we are. They don't always know. The best thing to do is take responsibility of your own life. Determine your own therapy. Take control, because it's too easy to let someone else do it for you. You don't have to be a number. Pull out the Bob Marley CD and let people see that you are an individual! It makes a difference.

Just before I moved out west, I had lunch with my friend Rita. At the end of our meal, we received fortune cookies.

"All this hard work will pay off," was my fortune.

Sometimes we don't think there will ever be an end in sight. That's when you have to push the hardest. Keeping positive people around you gives you that extra strength. In the end, however, only *you* can make you happy.

There are no guarantees for me, and that is difficult at times to live with. When I go to the doctor, I am reminded that I don't live a normal life. Some days, you feel as though you're living with a gun to your head, and you only hope that you won't suffer. And yet, they say that God gives you only what you can handle. I have made it so far. There's always that small fear whenever I have to meet with my doctor that I'll discover that the tumour is spreading, or they want to put me on chemo again. It happens. It's a part of my life. And if it gets too tough, I'll just grab a blanket, and Mission, go to a park and sit by the water . . . and get away from everything until it's time to face the music.

As soon as the appointment's over with, I'm flying high again. After all, ups and downs are what living is all about.

My name is Suzanne Giroux, and every day I cherish my gift, a chance for life.

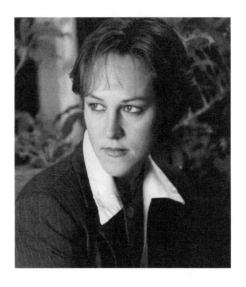

Robyn Burnett is a graduate of the UBC Creative Writing program, and since then has been writing in a variety of areas. At present, she has two screenplays optioned, and has just finished working on a short series of educational videos. For the past three years, she has volunteered with Camp Trillium, an organization that works with children with cancer and their families.